FITNESS PROFESSIONALS

THE FITNESS INSTRUCTOR'S
HANDBOOK

2nd edition

FITNESS PROFESSIONALS

THE FITNESS INSTRUCTOR'S
HANDBOOK

2nd edition

a complete guide to health and fitness

BLOOMSBURY · LONDON, NEW DELHI, NEW YORK, SYDNEY

First published 2007 by
A & C Black Publishers Ltd

Second edition © 2013

Published by Bloomsbury Publishing Plc
50 Bedford Square, London, WC1B 3DP
www.bloomsbury.com

Copyright © 2007, 2013

ISBN (print): 978 1 4081 7826 3
ISBN (e-pub): 978 1 4081 8169 0
ISBN (e-pdf): 978 1 4081 8168 3

The right of Morc Coulson to be identified as the author of this work has been asserted by him
in accordance with the Copyright, Designs and Patents Act 1988

A CIP catalogue record for this book is available from the British Library.

Note

It is always the responsibility of the individual to assess his or her own fitness
capability before participating in any training activity. Whilst every effort has been
made to ensure the content of this book is as technically accurate as possible,
neither the author nor the publishers can accept responsibility for any injury or
loss sustained as a result of the use of this material.

This book has been awarded 2 CPD points by the Register of Exercise
Professionals. REPs requires that all instructors regularly update their skills and
knowledge, which is evidenced by the recording of 24 CPD points every two
years with a minimum of 8 per year. If you already hold an industry qualification
you can answer the revision questions as part of your professional development.
For further information please visit the REPs website at www.exerciseregister.org.

Text and cover design by James Watson
Cover photograph © Shutterstock
Inside photographs courtesy of © Grant Pritchard and Chris Heron
All illustrations by Jeff Edwards with the exception of the following: pp. 6, 10, 18, 47, 75, 76, 77, 132, 133, 201,
204 and 223 by David Gardner

This book is produced using paper that is made from wood grown in managed, sustainable forests.
It is natural, renewable and recyclable. The logging and manufacturing processes conform to the
environmental regulations of the country of origin.

Typeset in Baskerville by seagulls.net
Printed and bound in China by C&C Offset Printing Co

10 9 8 7 6 5 4 3 2 1

CONTENTS

FOREWORD

Knowledge and support have helped many a top athlete over the years, not just physiologically but from a psychological, rehabilitational and medical perspective. It is common for individual athletes to use specifically designed programmes to train at the correct intensity, in the correct frame of mind and with nutritional advice that enables optimum recovery. There are also many recreational health and fitness participants who could benefit in many ways from support given by suitably qualified people. *The Fitness Instructor's Handbook* offers a comprehensive guide to the theory and practical application of health and fitness knowledge, linked closely to national occupational standards in this area. It is hoped that this book might help to develop a culture of education in health and fitness, not just for the benefit of the coach or instructor but for the entire population.

Steve Cram MBE and BBC TV Sports Personality of the Year 1983

PREFACE

This book has been written for a wide audience, such as those who have an interest in health and fitness and sport, or as a reference guide for individuals who, both now and in the future, may be involved in prescribing gym-based cardiovascular and resistance exercise to clients who are referred to as 'apparently healthy'. The main objective of the book is to address the underpinning knowledge requirement related to gym qualifications in the health and fitness industry, and show how that knowledge can be applied in a practical environment. It was a conscious decision to closely relate the book to health and fitness qualification requirements for two main reasons: firstly, to provide a comprehensive textbook that could help to promote the professionalism of the industry and secondly, there is a sparsity of textbooks in this country which comprehensively cover health and fitness knowledge criteria.

The chapter topics have been selected to provide a complete coverage of the required knowledge content for the 'Instructing Exercise and Fitness' qualification at Level 2 and the 'Instructing Physical Activity and Exercise' qualification at Level 3 (see Introduction). At the start of each chapter are the criteria related to Level 2 and 3 and the objectives to be addressed. At the end of the chapter you will find revision questions relating only to that particular chapter. Answers to these can be found at the back of the book, with space for revision notes. Each chapter also contains a list of further reading for those who would like to pursue the topic in more depth.

ACKNOWLEDGEMENTS

I would like to sincerely thank all who contributed in any way to the development and writing of this book. A big thank you goes out to Skills active and REPs for their continuing endeavours in trying to professionalise and bridge the gap between the Health and Fitness industry and academia and to the many training organisations who are actively embracing this philosophy.

Finally, many thanks to Sarah Cole, Editor at Bloomsbury, for her meticulous approach and co-ordination of the whole process.

INTRODUCTION

Since 2003 the government has been committed to the development of the nation's skills and in particular the education and training provision to address the nation's skills gaps and shortages. In order to facilitate this intention, organisations such as the **Fitness Industry Association** (FIA) and **SkillsActive** have taken a lead role.

The FIA was founded in 1991 to drive up participation and address concerns in the industry relating to safety and unfair codes of conduct. The fitness industry has since evolved and matured and, as the representative industry body, the FIA now works closely with Government to help deliver its public health targets and represent the interests of more than 2500 health and fitness organisations across the United Kingdom. FIA members include operators from the public and private sector, service/product suppliers to the industry, training providers, independent professionals and affiliated bodies. Members receive a variety of tailored, business-enhancing products and services specifically designed to support their particular business model or work.

The FIA's primary goal is to get more people, more active, more often. This is primarily achieved by developing and running high profile programmes designed to encourage people who are not regularly active to visit members' facilities. The FIA is also working on a regulated Code of Practice to replace its current voluntary Code.

SkillsActive is licensed by government as the Sector Skills Council for Active Leisure and Learning. Charged by employers, SkillsActive leads the skills and productivity drive across the sport and recreation, health and fitness, outdoors, playwork, and caravan industries – known as the active leisure and learning sector. SkillsActive work with health and fitness professionals across the United Kingdom to ensure the workforce is appropriately skilled and qualified. This includes working with higher and further education to develop qualification frameworks for new qualifications to enable graduates to leave college or university with industry-recognised vocational qualifications. The Register of Exercise Professionals (REPs) has also been set up to help safeguard and to promote the health and interests of people who are using the services of exercise and fitness instructors, teachers and trainers. REPs use a process of self-regulation that recognises industry-based qualifications, practical competency, and requires fitness professionals to work to a Code of Ethical Practice within the framework of National Occupational Standards that have been developed by SkillsActive. Qualifications needed to gain entry to the Register are closely aligned with National Occupational Standards. Below is an overview of the Level 2 and Level 3 qualification structures that provide entry onto the register.

Note: There is a Level 4 but the knowledge specific to this is not covered within this book.

Level 2 – Instructing Exercise and Fitness

There are four categories from which to gain entry to Level 2 of the exercise register: Gym, Exercise to Music, Aqua and Physical Activity for Children. Instructors may hold one or more of these categories. In order to gain an award at this level, individuals must successfully complete all of the mandatory units and one or more of the optional units as shown below. Individuals must also show competence of the core exercise and fitness knowledge criteria required at this level.

Note: Instructors must successfully complete all of the mandatory units below.

Level 2 Mandatory Units	
Unit code	Unit Description
A355	Reflect on and develop own practice in providing exercise and physical activity.
C22	Promote health safety and welfare in active leisure and recreation.
C316	Work with clients to help them to adhere to exercise and physical activity.

Note: Instructors may hold one or more optional units.

Level 2 Optional Units	
Gym	
D451	Plan and prepare a gym-based exercise.
D452	Instruct and supervise gym-based exercise.
Exercise to Music	
D453	Plan and prepare group exercise to music.
D454	Instruct group exercise to music.
Aqua	
D455	Plan and prepare water-based exercise.
D456	Instruct water-based exercise.
Physical activity for children	
D457	Plan health related exercise and physical activity for children.
D458	Instruct children in health related exercise and physical activity.

Level 3 – Instructing Physical Activity

There are four categories at Level 3 of the exercise register. Fitness Instructor/Personal Trainer, Advanced Exercise to Music, Exercise Referral and EMDP (exercise, music and dance partnership)/Yoga/Pilates. In order to gain an award at this level, individuals must successfully complete all of the units related to one or more of the areas as shown below. Individuals must also show competence of the core exercise and fitness knowledge required at this level.

Note: Instructors must display knowledge in all of the areas shown below.

Knowledge area	
1	Behaviour Change
2	Anatomy
3	Functional Kinesiology
4	Energy Systems
5	Concepts and Components of Fitness

Note: Instructors must successfully complete all of the units in one of more of the areas below:

Level 3 Units	
Personal trainer	
D460	Design, manage and adapt a personal training programme with clients.
D461	Deliver exercise and physical activity as part of a personal training programme.
D462	Apply the principles of nutrition to support client goals as part of an exercise and physical activity programme.
Exercise referral	
D463	Design, manage and adapt a physical activity programme with referred patients.
D464	Instruct exercise and physical activity with referred patients.
Advanced exercise to music	
D470	Design, manage and adapt an exercise to music programme incorporating advanced teaching strategies.
D471	Deliver exercise to music sessions incorporating advanced teaching strategies.
EMDP/Yoga/Pilates	
D465	Design, manage and adapt a mat Pilates programme.
D466	Instruct mat Pilates sessions.

Having gained a Level 2 or Level 3 award there are additional categories that can be accessed as shown below.

Additional Categories (accessed from either Level 2 or 3)	
Older adults	
D467	Adapt a physical activity programme to the needs of older adults.
Disability	
D468	Adapt a physical activity programme to the needs of disabled clients.
Ante/post natal	
D469	Adapt a physical activity programme to the needs of ante and postnatal clients.

Essentially, Level 2 and 3 instructors can only work on a one-to-one basis with apparently healthy individuals (unless they hold a relevant qualification) for whom screening has been carried out (see Chapter 11), however, they may on occasion allow appropriately screened and asymptomatic* special population** individuals to take part in mainstream studio, aqua or gym exercise sessions. Instructors must be aware, however, that if this becomes regular then they must endeavour to become qualified in the appropriate area.

* Asymptomatic is the term used to denote the absence of any specified key symptoms of disease identified in screening.

** Special population clients are those deemed by SkillsActive to include the following;
• 14–16-year-old people
• Disabled people
• Older people (50+)
• Ante- and post-natal women

Once accepted onto the register, instructors must continue their personal development by attending a minimum number of hours each year in the format of further qualifications, workshops, seminars or conferences, which have been accredited by REPs, in order to remain on the register. This is known as 'continuing professional development' or CPD. It is important that instructors regularly reflect on their performance and knowledge base in order to identify any training needs so that they provide the best possible advice for clients. This can be done by way of appraisal with other industry professionals with a view to developing a personal action plan with regards to CPD training.

Note: Instructors on the register can purchase public liability insurance but they must ensure that their insurance covers the populations that they are qualified to instruct.

Duty of Care (law of tort in England or delict in Scotland)

Any instructor working in the industry must be aware that they have a duty of care towards all individuals in that they must exercise a reasonable level of care in order to avoid injury to individuals and their property. This includes a duty of care towards vulnerable adults or clients that instructors are qualified to work with.

Note: A vulnerable adult is defined by the UK government as 'a person aged 18 years or over who is in receipt or need of community care services by reason of mental or other disability age or illness and who is or unable to take care of themselves or protect themselves against significant harm or exploitation'. A vulnerable client is someone undergoing a 'special' physiological lifespan process that puts them at a greater risk of an exercise related event (e.g. childhood, ageing, ante- and post-natal).

THEORETICAL KNOWLEDGE FOR HEALTH AND FITNESS

Part 1 of this book addresses the theoretical knowledge required for Level 2 and 3 Health Trainers within the Health and Fitness Industry. Each chapter provides example questions that are typical of Industry Standard Level 2 and 3 questions provided by accredited centres for the delivery of recognised qualifications. Part 1 also provides a list of recommended reading for each chapter should the reader wish to gain a more in-depth knowledge of the relevant topic area.

THE SKELETAL SYSTEM

OBJECTIVES

After completing this chapter, you will be able to:

1 Describe the structure of bone, in particular long bones.

2 Classify bones and give examples of each type.

3 Describe the process of bone growth, in particular within long bones.

4 Discuss the factors that can affect bone density.

5 Explain the effects of exercise on bone.

6 Describe the structure and list the functions of the skeleton.

7 Identify the major bones in the body.

8 Describe the structure and list the functions of the vertebral column.

9 Describe the structure and function of vertebral and intervertebral discs.

10 Describe the range of motion available at the spine.

11 Describe common postural definitions and list a range of common injuries associated with the spine.

Level 2: Instructing Exercise and Fitness Knowledge

Basic Anatomy and Physiology

■ The structure and function of the skeleton; structure and range of movement of the spine; bone growth.

■ The long- and short-term effects of exercise on bone.

Level 3: Instructing Physical Activity and Exercise Knowledge

Anatomy: Bones

■ Five types of bone:
 • Structure and proportion of compact/cancellous bone
 • Typical location/role within the body

- Structure of a long bone:
  - Diaphysis, epiphysis, epiphyseal plate, periosteum, medullary cavity, cartilage, compact bone, cancellous bone
  - Susceptibility to breakage/damage – epiphysis vs diaphysis
- Growth of a long bone:
  - The ossification process: pre-natal through childhood to adulthood
  - The role of osteoblasts and osteoclasts
  - Hormonal regulation of bone growth
  - Key nutrients in bone growth
  - Calcium regulation
  - Bone remodelling
  - Osteoporosis
- Names of all major bones:
  - Articulations and joint movements
  - Muscle attachment sites
- The skeletal system (axial and appendicular skeleton):
  - Structure and function of each part
- Structure of the spine; postural deviation:
  - Five curves of the skeleton
  - Number and structure of vertebrae in each section
  - The vertebral foramen
  - Structure and function of vertebral discs
  - Facet joints
  - Kyphosis, lordosis and scoliosis
  - Neutral spine
- The range of medical conditions common in back pain patients that may be aggravated by physical activity or lead to injury.

Introduction

This chapter deals with the anatomical systems of the body, in particular the formation of bone and the skeletal system from the perspective of structure and function, as well as the effects of exercise on these systems. Within the National Occupational Standards framework, Level 2 and 3 instructors should be able to identify the components of the skeletal system and describe their functions, as well as describe how exercise can impact on bone growth.

Later chapters provide physiological and biomechanical principles that, together with the anatomical knowledge covered in this chapter, will provide fitness instructors with the understanding and ability to design appropriate exercise programmes for apparently healthy individuals and to understand the effects of various types of exercise on the human body.

Common anatomical terms

As the first part of this book is concerned with the anatomy of the human body, it is useful to understand the terms used to describe it. When using anatomical terms, the body is assumed to be in a position where the arms are resting by the sides of the body with the palms facing forward, with a theoretical line drawn down the centre of the body. When the limbs move, the movement is described in reference to this line. Table 1.1 contains some common anatomical terms and their description.

Table 1.1	Common anatomical terms
Term	Description
Anterior	Front
Posterior	Back
Medial	Toward the mid-line
Lateral	Away from the mid-line
Superior	Upper
Inferior	Lower
Proximal	Near to
Distal	Away from
Prone	Facing down
Supine	Facing up

Bone

Bone structure

Bone is classified as a calcified connective tissue and, when it is fully developed, is the hardest tissue in the body. In a typical bone there are two types of bone tissue: *compact* and *cancellous*.

Compact bone

Compact bone is also known as *cortical* bone. It has a hard outer layer that provides a strong structure called the *cortex*, which provides protection and support to help resist stresses imposed during movement and weight-bearing activities. It is often assumed that compact bone is solid, but this is not the case: it contains a series of canals through which blood and lymph vessels and nerves pass. This series of canals gives compact bone greater strength than if the bone was completely solid, as the canal systems are aligned in the same direction along the lines of stress of each bone, helping to resist fracture.

Cancellous bone

Cancellous bone is otherwise known as *trabecular* bone. Within cancellous bone there is a 'spongy' structure that contains red bone marrow, which is where blood cells are made. This type of bone also contains a series of canals that are larger than those in compact bone as the red bone marrow needs to get a rich blood supply to produce red blood cells.

A double layer of tough, dense collagen fibres about the thickness of a nail, called the *periosteum*, covers most of the surface of bones. It provides attachment for tendons and ligaments and gives protection to the bone.

Classification of bones

Bones are often classified according to their formation and shape. The shape of a bone can sometimes help to identify the role it has in the body. Bone is normally classified into the five groups below (see also Fig. 1.1).

1. Long bones

Long bones are found mainly in the limbs and comprise a shaft with two extremities. The shaft is known as the *diaphysis* and the extremities are known as the *epiphyses*. Just before each epiphysis is a region known as the growth plate or *epiphyseal cartilage*. This is the region in the bone at which growth occurs; when growth finally stops in adulthood the epiphyseal cartilage becomes fully developed bone. Fatty yellow bone marrow is found within the central part of the long bone known as the *medullary canal*. Long bones are attached to muscles that can pull and create movement, so they act as levers to provide locomotion for the body. The femur and humerus are examples of long bones.

2. Short bones

Short bones are designed mainly for lightness and strength. They are usually cube-shaped and are mainly spongy (cancellous) bone with a thin outer layer of compact bone. Examples of short bones are the carpals (wrist) and tarsals (ankle).

3. Flat bones

Flat bones are spongy (cancellous) bones sandwiched between two layers of compact bone. They either give protection, such as in the skull, or provide a large area for muscle attachment, such as in the pelvis.

Fig. 1.1   Examples of the different types of bone in the body

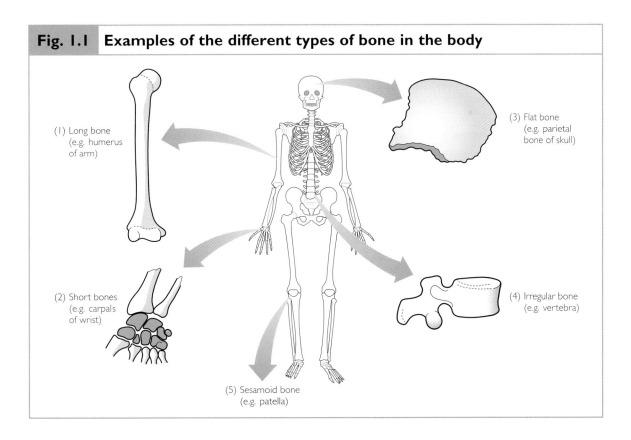

(1) Long bone (e.g. humerus of arm)

(2) Short bones (e.g. carpals of wrist)

(3) Flat bone (e.g. parietal bone of skull)

(4) Irregular bone (e.g. vertebra)

(5) Sesamoid bone (e.g. patella)

4. Irregular bones

Irregular bones usually have bony projections for the purpose of muscle attachment. The vertebrae (bones of the spine) are examples of irregular bones.

5. Sesamoid bones

Sesamoid bones are seed-like bones, normally the size of a pea, that are developed within the tendon of a muscle, such as the patella in the knee joint. Sesamoid bones usually protect tendons from excessive wear and tear. They can also change the direction of pull of a tendon to increase the mechanical advantage at a joint in which the tendon crosses.

TASK

Fig. 1.1 shows examples of the five types of bone and where they can be found in the body. Try to identify all of the bones in the skeleton and assign them to one of the five classifications.

Bone growth

Bone growth in humans begins at birth and is not complete until about the 25th year but can, in some cases, be complete around the age of 18. Bones start out in the body as tissues known as cartilage, membrane and tendon until a process called *ossification* (*oss* meaning bone and *fication* meaning to make) gradually replaces these tissues with bone. Certain hormones released within the body, such as *growth hormone*, testosterone, oestrogen and calcitonin, help to regulate and control bone development.

Long bones, such as those in the limbs, grow in length at the epiphyseal or growth plate, which is the region near the end of the diaphysis or shaft of the bone (see Fig. 1.2). The ends, or epiphyses, of long bones are enlarged and are covered in a tissue called hyaline cartilage (see page 74), which provides protection for the end of the bone.

TASK

Draw and label the parts of a typical long bone and list the functions of each part.

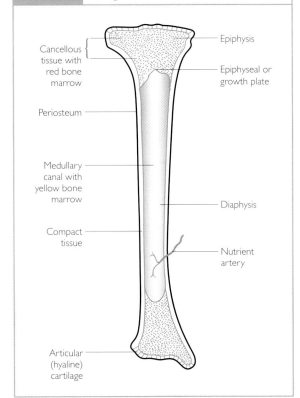

Fig. 1.2 The structure of a typical long bone

- Epiphysis
- Epiphyseal or growth plate
- Cancellous tissue with red bone marrow
- Periosteum
- Medullary canal with yellow bone marrow
- Compact tissue
- Diaphysis
- Nutrient artery
- Articular (hyaline) cartilage

Bone tissue contains several types of cell. An *osteocyte* is the main cell of a fully developed bone. Two other types of bone cell, *osteoblasts* and *osteoclasts*, are responsible for building and modelling the bone in which they are located. Osteoblasts are bone-building cells that are involved in the formation of bone; osteoclasts are very large bone-modelling cells that can break down bone formation by digesting protein and minerals, making the bone less dense and therefore weaker. Throughout life, if homeostasis is achieved, then osteoblasts and osteoclasts work together to keep bone at the optimum thickness. If homeostasis is disrupted, it is possible that one type of bone cell can dominate, resulting in either a thickening or weakening of the bone.

Ossification can start as early as in the womb, where osteoblasts secrete protein (primarily collagen) to initiate the process of calcification by forming a meshwork called the *bone matrix*. Osteoblasts get trapped in the matrix and become osteocytes (main bone cells) as the matrix calcifies and hardens. Other osteoblasts then work outwards to increase the length of the bone. At the same time, osteoclasts work to remove excess bone and prevent it from becoming too thick. Osteoblasts and osteoclasts work together at the epiphyses of the bone to form an epiphyseal plate, which is responsible for bone growth. This activity is controlled by many hormones at different stages throughout life; one of the most important is growth hormone, which is secreted by the *pituitary gland*.

During growth, the epiphyseal plate is just a layer of hyaline cartilage. When bones stop growing in length (usually between the ages of 18 and 25) the hyaline cartilage at the epiphyseal plate is replaced by bone. Even though bones do not grow in length after this stage, they can continue to grow in diameter throughout life.

Factors affecting bone growth

Age, lack of weight-bearing activity, smoking and alcoholism can all lead to a loss of calcium and bone marrow. The cancellous part of the bone, therefore, becomes less dense, making the bone weaker and slower to heal. A severe case of this condition is known as osteoporosis, which is more common in females (especially post-menopausal) than males: figures suggest that up to 50 per cent of post-menopausal women suffer from the condition. Even though it is thought that osteoporosis is not reversible, many studies have shown that exercise can slow down the rate at which osteoporosis occurs – the pull of muscles on bone and the effects of gravity can lead to an increase in bone density (Baechle, 1994; Wilmore and Costhill, 2004). It is therefore important that some type of resistance training be recommended to people with this condition, although care should be taken due to the risk of bone fracture or breaks.

NEED TO KNOW

The density of bone can be estimated using a technique known as dual-energy X-ray absorptiometry (DEXA). This technique, which involves a very low dose of photon radiation, can also be used to estimate body-fat percentage.

NEED TO KNOW

Other hormones that influence bone growth include thyroxine, testosterone, oestrogen, calcitonin and parathormone.

Diet also has an impact on bone growth and strength. Almost half the content of bone is made up of the minerals calcium and phosphorous. Calcium is always present in the blood as it has many functions in the body, for example, it is required for muscle contraction and bone formation (normal blood calcium levels are 9–11 mg per 100 ml of blood). If blood calcium levels fall, osteoclasts will break down bone to release calcium into the bloodstream. Therefore, a diet low in calcium can make the bones weaker. About 80 per cent of the phosphorous in the body is found in and is responsible for the formation of bones and teeth. It also plays an important part in muscle contraction. Dietary sources include dairy products, meat, fish and beans. Finally, vitamins C and D are also important in the process of bone growth: vitamin C is used in the laying down of collagen to form connective tissue, such as in bone formation, while vitamin D is essential for the absorption of calcium and phosphorous from the intestine.

The effects of exercise on bone

Physical activity has been shown to stimulate osteoblasts to secrete protein and initiate the bone-building process as a result of placing force on the bone. This is referred to as the *minimal essential strain.* The exact amount of activity required to start this process is unknown, but is thought to be equivalent to one-tenth of the force required to fracture the bone. Forces placed on the bone below this threshold are believed to have no effect. Many studies have also shown a correlation between bone density and the strength of the attached musculature, so it appears that resistance training has a positive effect on bone density. However, the formation of new

bone is relatively slow compared to the rapid loss of bone mineral content as a result of immobility or reduced loading, especially following a period of bed-rest.

NEED TO KNOW

In general terms, an increase or decrease in muscle strength will result in a corresponding increase or decrease in bone density.

Short-term effects

There are no actual short-term effects of exercise on the bones; instead, exercise initiates the long-term process described below.

Long-term effects

Placing stress on the bones by engaging in weight-bearing exercise is thought to result in the bone tissue becoming stronger over a period of time. However, care must be taken not to place too much stress or high impact on the bones of children who have not fully matured, as this can result in damage to the epiphyseal plate.

Exactly how placing stress on the bones results in stronger bone tissue is still a case for debate. However, it is commonly agreed that resistance or impact exercise places stress on the bones that stimulate this mechanism. It is recommended that adolescents and young adults should engage in some sort of weight-bearing activity to help this process occur, but, as stated above, the amount of stress must be limited.

It is also recommended that older adults engage in some sort of bone-stressing exercise, because as we get older the amount of calcium taken out of the bones is greater than the amount of calcium taken in by the bones. This is due to the fact that activity levels and dietary intake of calcium and phosphorous usually reduces, while in post-menopausal women a reduction in hormone levels disrupts the activity of osteoblasts. In the long term, this makes the bones less dense and therefore weaker.

NEED TO KNOW

Astronauts in space can lose as much as 1 per cent of bone mass per week due to the lack of gravity.

The skeleton

Structure and functions of the skeleton

The human skeleton contains approximately 206 bones and consists of two parts: the *axial skeleton*, which comprises the skull, the vertebral column (backbone), the ribs and the sternum; and the *appendicular skeleton* (*appendic* meaning 'to hang on to'), which comprises the shoulder and pelvic girdles and the upper and lower limbs (see Fig. 1.3). The skeleton as a whole has many important functions, including:

- Providing a framework and shape for the body: the size and shape of the skeleton can determine a person's shape (see page 165).
- Protecting the vital organs: for example, the ribcage protects the heart and lungs.

Table 1.2	The bones of the shoulder girdle	
Bone	Landmark	Description
Scapula	Acromion process	• Projection over the shoulder joint • Site of muscular attachment • Articulates with the clavicle
	Coracoid process	• Projection on the anterior aspect of scapula • Site of attachment for the short head of the biceps
	Spine of the scapula	• Large ridge extending from the acromion process across the posterior surface of the scapula to the medial border of the scapula
	Glenoid fossa	• Shallow depression where the humerus articulates with the scapula
Clavicle	Acromial end	• Articulates with acromion process of the scapula
	Sternal end	• Articulates with the manubrium of the sternum

Fig. 1.3 The bones of (a) the axial and (b) the appendicular skeleton

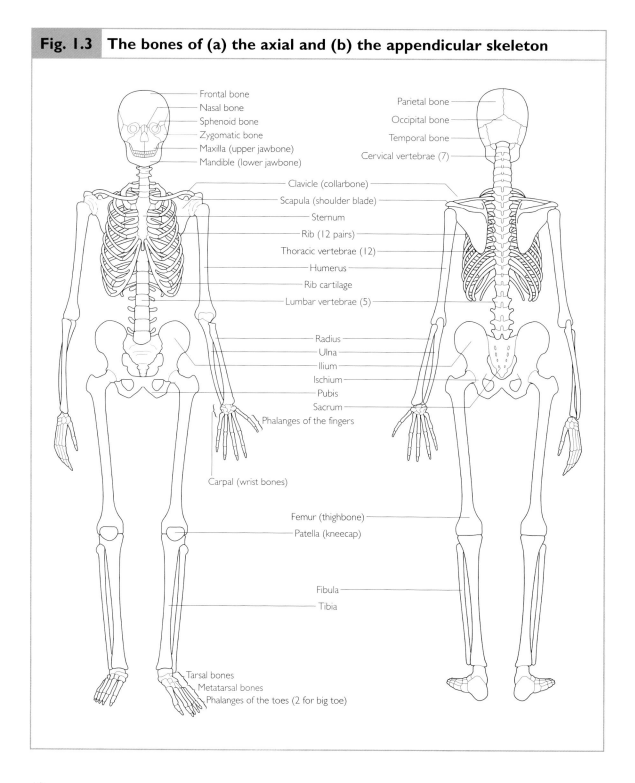

Frontal bone
Nasal bone
Sphenoid bone
Zygomatic bone
Maxilla (upper jawbone)
Mandible (lower jawbone)

Parietal bone
Occipital bone
Temporal bone
Cervical vertebrae (7)

Clavicle (collarbone)
Scapula (shoulder blade)
Sternum
Rib (12 pairs)
Thoracic vertebrae (12)
Humerus
Rib cartilage
Lumbar vertebrae (5)

Radius
Ulna
Ilium
Ischium
Pubis
Sacrum
Phalanges of the fingers

Carpal (wrist bones)

Femur (thighbone)
Patella (kneecap)

Fibula
Tibia

Tarsal bones
Metatarsal bones
Phalanges of the toes (2 for big toe)

- Acting as levers for movement on which muscles act. When muscles contract they draw together and, as the ends of muscles are normally attached to bones, one attachment will move towards the other.
- Providing surfaces for the attachment of muscles (via tendons) and ligaments.
- Producing red and white blood cells and platelets. This is the function of the cancellous or 'spongy' bone.
- Storing minerals such as calcium, phosphorus, potassium and sodium.

It is important that health and fitness instructors are familiar with the names and locations of the bones in the body as, together with the muscles, they provide movement and locomotion.

The bones of the shoulder (pectoral) girdle

See Table 1.2 and Fig. 1.4. The shoulder or pectoral girdle attaches the arms to the body, or, in other words, the upper limbs to the axial skeleton. It consists of a *scapula* (shoulder blade) and *clavicle* (collar bone) on each side of the body. The scapula has a socket called the *glenoid fossa* or *cavity*, which articulates (joins) with the upper arm (*humerus*) to form the shoulder joint. This

is a shallow joint that allows for a large degree of mobility at the expense of stability. The most lateral point of the scapula is called the *acromion process*, which articulates with the clavicle to form the acromioclavicular joint. The distance between the two acromion processes is called the *biacromial distance*.

The bones of the upper and lower arm

See Table 1.3 and Fig. 1.5. The humerus is the bone of the upper arm that, along with the glenoid fossa of the scapula, makes the shoulder joint. The distal (far) end of the humerus articulates with the two bones of the lower arm or forearm (with the *radius* at the *capitulum* and with the *ulna* at the *trochlear*) to form the elbow joint.

The bones of the hand and wrist

See Table 1.4 and Fig. 1.6. The eight short bones located in the wrist are known collectively as the *carpals*. The bones are held together tightly by ligaments (see pages 74–7) and have only a small degree of movement. The carpal bones articulate with the ulna and radius to form the wrist joint. At their furthest point, the carpals

Fig. 1.4 Bones of the shoulder girdle

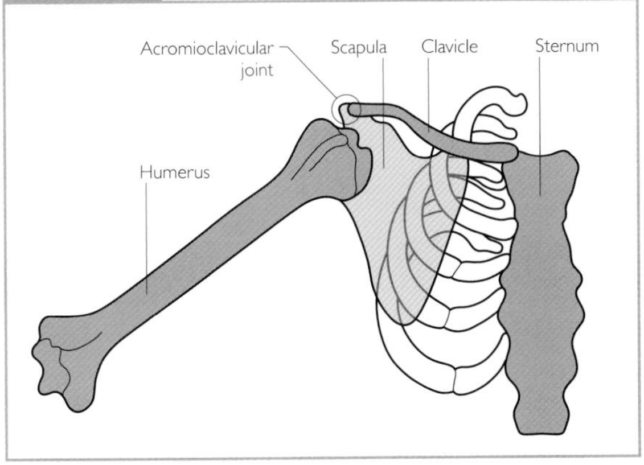

Acromioclavicular joint · Scapula · Clavicle · Sternum · Humerus

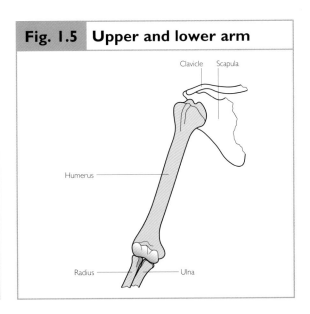

Fig. 1.5 Upper and lower arm

Clavicle · Scapula · Humerus · Radius · Ulna

Table 1.3	The bones of the upper and lower arm	
Bone	**Landmark**	**Description**
Humerus	Head	• Smooth, round proximal surface that articulates with the glenoid fossa of the scapula
	Humeral condyles (capitulum and trochlear)	• Articular surfaces on the medial and lateral sides of the distal humerus • Capitulum articulates with the head of the radius • Trochlear articulates with the trochlear notch on the ulna
Ulna	Olecranon process	• Process at the proximal end of the ulna • Point of the elbow • Attachment point for the posterior arm muscles
	Head	• Small, partially rounded distal end that articulates with the radius and wrist bones
Radius	Head	• Proximal, drum-shaped end • Articulates with the capitulum of the humerus and the radial notch of the ulna

Table 1.4	The bones of the hand and wrist	
Bone	**Landmark**	**Description**
Carpals	Triquetrum Trapezoid Trapezium Hamate Lunate Capitate Pisiform Scaphoid	• Articulate with the radius and ulna at the proximal side and with the metacarpals at the distal side
Metacarpals		• Short bones located within the palm
Phalanges	Proximal, medial and distal	• Proximal, medial and distal sections allow individual movement for dexterity

articulate with five bones in the palm of the hand called the *metacarpals* (*meta* meaning 'beyond'). The metacarpals then articulate with the fingers or *phalanges*, each of which comprises proximal (near), medial (middle) and distal (far) sections, except for the thumb, which has only two sections.

Fig. 1.6	**Bones of the hand and the wrist**

Scaphoid — Radius
Trapezoid — Ulna
Lunate
Pisiform
Trapezium — Triquetrum
Hamate
Metacarpals
Capitate — Phalanges

The bones of the pelvic girdle

See Table 1.5 and Fig. 1.7. The pelvic girdle provides a strong base to which the axial skeleton attaches via the vertebral column, making a fused joint with the *sacrum*. This is called the *sacroiliac joint*. On each side of the pelvis is a socket called the *acetabulum*, which forms a joint with the femur of the upper leg. This is a deep socket that provides a high degree of stability, but has less mobility than the shoulder girdle. The pelvic girdle protects the internal organs,

Fig. 1.7	**Bones of the pelvic girdle**

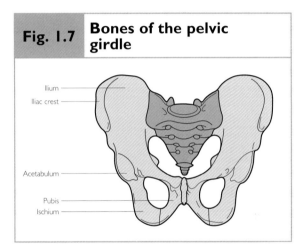

Ilium
Iliac crest
Acetabulum
Pubis
Ischium

Table 1.5	The bones of the pelvic girdle	
Bone	Landmark	Description
Ilium		• Large, flat, superior wing-like portion of the pelvis
	Iliac crest	• Large ridge on the superior part of the ilium
Ischium		• Posterior, inferior portion of the pelvis
Pubis		• Anterior, inferior portion of the pelvis
	Acetabulum	• Depression into which the head of the femur articulates

and in women also provides protection for the foetus during pregnancy. The distance between the two most lateral points is known as the *bicristal distance* and is usually greater in females than in males.

The bones of the upper and lower leg

See Table 1.6 and Fig. 1.8. The *femur* (thigh bone) is a long bone in the upper leg and is the longest bone in the body. At the top or head of the femur is a ball-shaped part of the bone that

Table 1.6 The bones of the upper and lower leg		
Bone	Landmark	Description
Femur	Head	• Articulates with the acetabulum of the pelvis
	Greater trochanter	• Large process on the lateral side of the proximal end of bone, to which the gluteal muscles attach
	Condyles	• Rounded medial and lateral smooth articular surfaces where the femur articulates with the tibia
	Intercondylar fossa	• Deep groove between the condyles where the cruciate ligaments attach
	Epicondyles	• Small medial and lateral ridges where the muscles attach
Tibia	Condyles	• Flat, smooth medial and lateral surfaces with which the femur articulates
	Intercondylar eminence	• Crest between the condyles where the cruciate ligaments attach
	Tibial tuberosity	• Knot on the anterior, proximal surface where the patellar ligament attaches
	Medial malleolus	• Large process of the distal, medial aspect of the bone
Fibula	Head	• Proximal enlargement • Articulates with the lateral aspect of the proximal tibia
	Lateral malleolus	• Enlargement on the distal, lateral aspect of the bone
Patella		• Large sesamoid bone in the tendon of the quadriceps muscles of the anterior thigh

articulates with the socket (*acetabulum*) of the pelvis to form the hip joint. At the bottom of the femur are two smooth, rounded surfaces that articulate with the *tibia* to form the *tibiofemoral* or knee joint. Each end of the femur is covered in hyaline cartilage (see page 74).

At the front of the knee joint is a small, triangular sesamoid bone called the *patella* (meaning 'little dish'), which is otherwise known as the knee cap. The patella is located within a band of tendon (see pages 77–8) and glides over the groove on the end of the femur as the knee joint flexes and extends. This is known as the *patellofemoral joint.*

The *tibia* is the main weight-bearing bone in the lower leg and is sometimes known as the shin bone. The top of the tibia is a broad flat surface that articulates with the femur to form the knee joint. The bottom of the tibia articulates with one of the tarsal bones in the ankle, called the *talus*, to form the ankle joint. The *fibula* is a long bone that runs down the lateral side of the tibia and makes a fibrous joint (see page 26) at both ends with the tibia.

The bones of the foot and ankle

See Table 1.7 and Fig. 1.9. The seven short bones in the back section of the foot are collectively known as the *tarsals*. The *calcaneus* is the largest of the tarsal bones and is otherwise known as the heel bone. The *talus* is most superior and articulates with the tibia to form the ankle joint. As with the carpals, the tarsal bones are held together tightly by ligaments (see pages 75–6) and have only a small degree of movement.

In the mid-foot are five bones known as the *metatarsals* that articulate with the toes, which, like the fingers, are known as *phalanges*. Again, like the fingers, each phalange except for the big toe has three sections: the proximal (nearest), medial (middle) and distal (farthest) phalanges.

Fig. 1.8	Bones of upper and lower leg

Labels: Greater trochanter, Head, Neck, Lesser trochanter, Shaft, **Femur**, Lateral epicondyle, **Knee**, Patella (knee cap), Medial epicondyle, **Fibula**, **Tibia**

Fig. 1.9	Bones of the foot and ankle

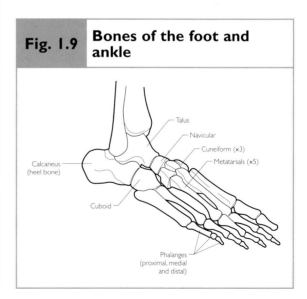

Labels: Talus, Navicular, Cuneiform (×3), Metatarsals (×5), Calcaneus (heel bone), Cuboid, Phalanges (proximal, medial and distal)

Table 1.7	The bones of the foot and ankle	
Bone	Landmark	Description
Tarsals	Calcaneus talus Cuboid Cuneiform (x3) Navicular	The talus articulates with the tibia and fibula at the proximal side. The 3 cuneifrm bones and the cuboid articulate with the metatarsals at the distal side.
Metatarsals		Short bones located between the ankle joint and the mid-foot.
Phalanges	Proximal, medial and distal	Proximal, medial and distal sections to allow individual movement and flexibility.

The structure and functions of the vertebral column

The spine, otherwise known as the vertebral column or backbone, consists of 24 separate moveable bones called *vertebrae* (separated by *intervertebral discs*) and nine fused bones. The moveable bones are in three regions – *cervical, thoracic* and *lumbar* – and the fused bones are in two regions – *sacrum* and *coccyx* (see Fig. 1.10).

The spine is essentially a strong and flexible column that acts as a support system on which the limbs are able to move. Viewed from the side, the structure is curved. The thoracic and sacral regions of the spine are known as primary curves, while the cervical and lumbar regions are known as secondary curves. These curves increase the strength of the vertebral column and provide shock absorption during walking, running and jumping.

The top vertebra in the spine is known as the *atlas* and makes a joint with the skull. The bone underneath the atlas is called the *axis* and, along with the atlas, provides a pivot that enables the skull to rotate. The neck region of the spine, made up of seven bones, is known as the cervical region and allows a degree of movement for the head. Below this, in the upper part of the body, is the thoracic region of the spine, which comprises 12 bones. Here,

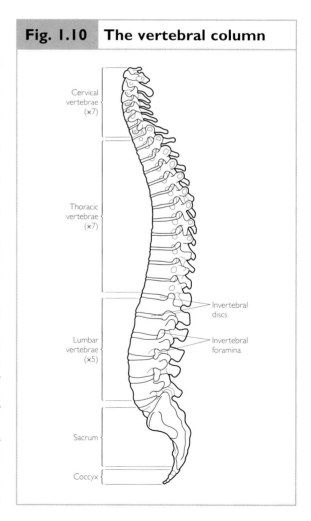

Fig. 1.10 The vertebral column

Cervical vertebrae (×7)

Thoracic vertebrae (×7)

Lumbar vertebrae (×5)

Sacrum

Coccyx

Invertebral discs

Invertebral foramina

movement is limited as the ribcage is attached to the spine in this region. Below this, in the lower part of the back, is the lumbar spine, made up of five bones. There is a wide range of movement available in this region, as this is the part of the spine from which the upper body bends forward and from side to side. The region of the spine known as the sacrum consists of five fused bones and is attached to the pelvis. Finally, the coccyx at the bottom of the spine is made up of four fused bones, but really serves no purpose.

As well as attaching the lower part of the body to the upper part, the spine serves many other functions in the body, including:

- Protecting the spinal cord – the main nerve stem from the brain, which runs through a hole (*foramen*) in the posterior part of each vertebra
- Providing access for blood and lymph vessels
- Allowing certain degrees of movement – each individual vertebra does not have much movement, but the spine as a unit does
- Providing support for the skull
- Providing attachment for the ribs and pelvic girdle (the part of the vertebral bodies where the ribs attach to the spine is known as a *facet*)
- Housing shock-absorbing discs

Vertebral bodies and intervertebral discs

The vertebrae in different regions of the spine can vary slightly in shape and size but essentially share the same features (see Fig. 1.11), especially between the second cervical vertebra and the fifth lumbar vertebra. Each vertebra usually has a disc-shaped body with several bony processes that extend from the back of the body, which allow for the attachment of muscles via tendons. At the ends of the bony processes are surfaces known as *facets* that are covered in smooth tissue called *articular cartilage*. The facets of one vertebra make a joint, known as a *zygapophyseal joint*, with the facets of the vertebrae

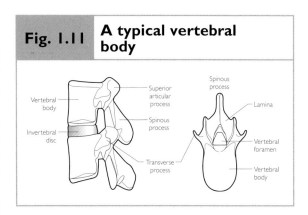

Fig. 1.11 A typical vertebral body

above and below. These joints are synovial (gliding) joints – lubricated with synovial fluid – that allow movement of the spine. The range of motion in each section of the spine mainly depends on the facet joints. The main body of a typical vertebra has an opening on the posterior side known as a *vertebral foramen*, which provides a protective channel through which the spinal cord can run. Nerves branching out from the spinal cord exit from gaps between each adjacent pair of vertebrae.

Between the bodies of adjacent vertebrae are *intervertebral discs* (see Fig. 1.11), which provide shock absorption for the spine. The outer layer of the disc, called the *annulus fibrosus* (annulus meaning 'ringlike'), is made of cartilaginous fibres and is very tough. The inner part of the disc is called the *nucleus pulposus* (pulposus meaning 'pulplike') and is made of a soft, viscous, fluid-like material that is very elastic.

Together with the vertebrae, the intervertebral discs provide strong joints in the spine that can withstand a certain amount of compression and stretching. However, it is possible for the outer layer of the disc (the annulus fibrosus) to be ruptured so that the inner part of the disc (the nucleus pulposus) protrudes. This is commonly known as a *slipped* or *herniated disc*. It is possible for the nucleus pulposus to exert pressure on a spinal nerve, causing pain either locally or along the length of the nerve.

The discs increase in thickness from the top to the bottom of the spine and can reduce in thickness throughout the day due to the effects of compression and lack of hydration. The discs can return to their original size overnight if hydrated, but due to the ageing process can degenerate and become thinner as we get older.

Range of movement of the vertebral column

The range of movement between each individual bone in the spine is limited because of the facet joints, as mentioned above. However, the spine as a whole is capable of a wide range of movement, including *flexion* (bending forward), *extension* (bending backward), *lateral flexion* or *extension* (bending to the side) and *rotation*. The spine has more movement in the cervical and lumbar regions than anywhere else. Flexion and extension of the spine occur mainly at the lower two lumbar vertebrae; however, there is a limited degree of rotation at the lumbar spine. Flexion and extension are limited in the thoracic spine due to the attachment of the ribs, but there is a reasonable amount of rotation.

Age can decrease the movement available in the spine; it is therefore recommended that mobilisation and flexibility exercises make up an important part of an overall exercise programme with older adults.

There are many published tables available that provide information about the ranges of motion available at the spine. However, the ranges of motion can differ depending on which author has published the tables; therefore, Table 1.8 shows a typical range of motion for movements of the spine that are common to the published ranges.

Postural definitions

The facet joints and intervertebral discs provide the spine with a certain amount of rigidity, but this is not an adequate amount of support to maintain posture at all times. The muscles provide a certain amount of support, as do the many ligaments that surround the spine (see fig 1.12). There are two main groups of ligaments related to the spine: the *intrasegmental* and the *intersegmental* ligaments. Like all ligaments, the spinal ligaments allow a certain degree of wanted movement, but are designed to prevent unwanted movement.

The small range of motion at the spine where none of the spinal ligaments are placed under any tension is known as the *neutral zone*. This is considered to be correct alignment or posture for the spine. Postural imbalances can occur where spinal ligaments have been stretched, where spinal muscles are weak or where there are mechanical dysfunctions. Common postural problems include *kyphosis*, *lordosis* and *scoliosis*.

NEED TO KNOW

The secondary cervical curve develops only after about the first three months of life and the lumbar curve after 12 to 18 months.

| Fig. 1.12 | **Typical spinous ligaments** |

Intertransverse ligament

Ligamentum flavum

Posterior longitudinal ligament

Facet capsulary ligament

Interspinous ligament

Anterior longitudinal ligament

Supraspinous ligament

Table 1.8	Typical range of motion associated with the spinal column
Movement	Range of motion
Flexion	Total range of 45–55 degrees, mainly at the lumbar region
Extension	Typically 20–35 degrees
Lateral flexion	Up to 60 degrees to either side of the midline, but reducing quickly with age
Rotation	Limited to only a few degrees in the lumbar spine

Kyphosis

This term is used to describe an excessive secondary curve of the thoracic region of the spine. People who suffer from this condition are usually very round-shouldered or hunched in appearance. The diagnosis can often be complicated, but common back-strengthening exercises for the trapezius and rhomboid muscles are normally advocated.

Note: During pregnancy there is likely to be a greater forward shift of centre of gravity which increases lordosis (curved lower back) and can contribute to kyphosis (rounded shoulders).

Lordosis

This term describes an excessive primary curve of the lumbar region of the spine. The condition is sometimes referred to as 'sway-back' and is often associated with an increase in abdominal weight, for example, in pregnancy or obesity. Core stabilisation techniques are usually prescribed, as the anterior spinal ligaments can be damaged by this type of posture.

Scoliosis

There are different types of scoliosis, but the term generally refers to a twisting or abnormal curvature of the spine. Scoliosis is normally associated with the thoracic or upper lumbar areas of the spine, although in some cases it can occur in the lower part of the lumbar region. Specific exercises are sometimes effective to rectify muscular imbalance, but these need to be prescribed by a qualified person. For the different types of scoliosis, see Table 1.9.

Common spinal injuries

The spine is a complex mechanical structure and is therefore susceptible to many possible injuries. Injuries can occur in relation to the vertebrae, the spinal ligaments, the intervertebral discs, the spinal muscle and tendons or associated spinal nerves.

Vertebral body injuries

Fractures

Fractures to the vertebral body can be caused as a result of an external blow, known as an *extrinsic* injury, or as a result of internal forces, known as an *intrinsic* injury.

Spondylolysis

This term refers to the degenerative destruction of the vertebral bodies. The term spondylosis usually refers to a different stage of the same condition.

Spondylolisthesis

This term is used in the case of anterior or posterior sliding of one vertebral body over

Table 1.9	Types of scoliosis
Scoliosis type	Description
Congenital	This type of congenital deformity is quite rare
Neuromuscular	Due to muscle weakness or imbalance, it is possible for the spine to be pulled to one side
Degenerative	Due to the ageing process, it is possible for the spine to develop scoliosis
Idiopathic	This type of scoliosis normally develops in adolescence and usually has no known cause

another. In some cases the stress placed on the vertebral body can cause it to fracture.

Ligament injuries

Ligament tissue has only a slight degree of elasticity as its main function is to provide support. If the movement of the spine takes one of the numerous ligaments of the spine beyond its individual elastic limit, it could result in damage to the ligament. Tears of the ligament are known as *sprains*, whereas the term *rupture* is used to describe a ligament that has completely snapped.

Disc injuries

The term *disc lesion* refers to an injury of the intervertebral discs. The most common is disc protrusion, where the inner part of the disc (nucleus pulposis) pushes through the outer part of the disc (annulus fibrosis), which can in turn make contact with nerves and cause pain (see also nerve injuries).

Muscle and tendon injuries

Many muscles attach to the spinal column via tendons. Both muscle and tendon tissue can only withstand a certain amount of force, after which injury can occur. As with ligaments, tears in muscle or tendon are known as strains, whereas the term rupture is used for a muscle or tendon that has completely snapped.

Nerve injuries

Nerves that protrude from the spinal column are sometimes disturbed by other structures, such as a protrusion from the intervertebral disc, a narrowing of the spinal foramen or just a muscular spasm. Whatever the cause, any disturbance of a nerve will cause pain. This pain can either be localised or radiate away from the cause of the disturbance. The pain is sometimes given a name that relates to the origin of the nerve that is disturbed; for example, sciatic pain radiates down the leg through the sciatic nerves.

NEED TO KNOW

In certain cases of overweight and obesity, centre of gravity can be displaced due to the large amount of adipose tissue which in turn can lead to stress on structures such as ligament and tendon causing postural deviation.

TASK

List the common spinal injuries and give a brief description of each.

EXAMPLE QUESTIONS

1.1 The radius bone is an example of which type of bone?
a) long bone
b) short bone
c) flat bone
d) irregular bone

1.2 The patella is an example of which type of bone?
a) long bone
b) short bone
c) flat bone
d) sesamoid bone

1.3 The scapula is an example of which type of bone?
a) long bone
b) short bone
c) flat bone
d) sesamoid bone

1.4 What is the name for the area near the end of a long bone where growth occurs?
a) diaphysis
b) epiphysis
c) periostium
d) cancellous

1.5 Which two regions of the spine are secondary curves?
a) cervical and thoracic
b) thoracic and lumbar
c) lumbar and cervical
d) thoracic and sacrum

EXAMPLE QUESTIONS cont.

1.6 In which region of the spine are the bones fused?

a) cervical

b) thoracic

c) lumbar

d) sacrum

1.7 Tendons attach to a layer of tissue covering a bone. What is this covering called?

a) osteoclast

b) diaphysis

c) epiphyseal plate

d) periostium

1.8 Cells in the bone that are responsible for bone-building are called what?

a) cancellous cells

b) osteoblast cells

c) osteoclast cells

d) ossification cells

1.9 Cells in the bone that are responsible for breaking down bone are called what?

a) cancellous cells

b) osteoblast cells

c) osteoclast cells

d) ossification cells

1.10 In terms of postural deviation, an excessive primary curve of the thoracic region of the spine is usually referred to by what name?

a) lordosis

b) scoliosis

c) flat back

d) kyphosis

EXAMPLE QUESTIONS cont.

1.11 In terms of postural deviation, an excessive secondary curve of the lumbar region of the spine is usually referred to by what name?

a) lordosis

b) scoliosis

c) flat back

d) kyphosis

1.12 In terms of postural deviation, twisting of the spine is usually referred to by what name?

a) lordosis

b) scoliosis

c) flat back

d) kyphosis

Further reading

Abrahams, P., Craven, J. and Lumley, J. (2011) *Illustrated Clinical Anatomy* (2nd ed.), Hodder Arnold

Baechle, R.T. (2008) *Essentials of Strength Training and Conditioning* (3rd ed.), Human Kinetics

Department of Health (2004) *At least 5 a week: Evidence on the impact of physical activity and its relationship to health.* London: Department of Health

Norkin, C.C. and White, D.J. (2003) *Measurement of Joint Motion: A guide to goniometry* (3rd ed.), F.A. Davis

Porter, S. (2002) *The Anatomy Workbook*, Butterworth Heinemann

Ross, J.S. and Wilson, J.W. (2006) *Anatomy and Physiology in Health and Illness* (10th ed.), Churchill Livingstone

Sewell, D., Watkins, P. and Griffin, M. (2005) *Sport and Exercise Science: An Introduction*, Hodder Arnold

Tortora, G.J. and Grabowski, S.R. (2005) *Principles of Anatomy and Physiology* (11th ed.), Wiley

Wilmore, J.H. and Costhill, D.L. (2007) *Physiology of Sport and Exercise* (5th ed.), Human Kinetics

NOTES

JOINTS

OBJECTIVES

After completing this chapter, you will be able to:

1 List the different classifications of joints and give examples of each.

2 Distinguish between different types of joints by relating to their range of movement.

3 List and give examples of the different types of synovial joints.

4 Identify the common movements within each type of synovial joint.

5 Identify the typical structures within a synovial joint.

6 List the short- and long-term effects on joints.

7 List the effects of pregnancy on joint stability.

Level 2: Instructing Exercise and Fitness Knowledge

Basic anatomy and physiology

- The structure and function of a synovial joint; ranges of movement of major synovial joints.

- The long- and short-term effects of exercise on synovial joints.

Level 3: Instructing Physical Activity and Exercise Knowledge

Anatomy: Joints

- Three types of joints (fibrous, cartilaginous, synovial)
  - The characteristics of each joint
  - Examples of each joint
  - Stability vs movement within each type of joint
- Structure of synovial joints
  - Ligaments, articular cartilage, joint cavity, synovial membrane, synovial fluid
  - Structure and movement potential/anatomical limitations of major joints (shoulder, hip, knee and elbow)
  - Different types of synovial joints and their movement potential

- Names of all major bones
  - Articulations and joint movements
  - Muscle attachment sites
- Joint actions (flexion, extension, hyperextension, adduction, abduction, elevation, depression, lateral flexion, horizontal flexion and extension, plantar flexion, dorsiflexion, internal and external rotation, circumduction, pronation, supination, eversion, inversion)

Introduction

This chapter deals with the anatomical system of the body, in particular the classification of joints within the skeletal system from a perspective of structure, function and the effects of exercise. Within the National Occupational Standards framework, Level 2 and 3 instructors should be able to list the classifications of joints and describe the common structures in each type of joint, as well as describe how exercise can affect joints.

Later chapters provide physiological and biomechanical principles that, together with the anatomical knowledge covered in this chapter, provide the instructor with the understanding and ability to design appropriate exercise programmes for apparently healthy individuals and to understand the effects of various types of exercise on the human body.

Basic types of joint

A simple definition of a joint is the articulation or place where two or more bones meet. In other words, a joint is the place where bones come together. Joints are normally classified according to their structure and function, and there are three broad types: *fibrous, cartilaginous* and *synovial.* Fibrous and cartilaginous joints contain connective tissue that binds bone together, whereas synovial joints have a fluid-filled capsule, but no connective tissue, binding the joint. Joints can also be classified according to their degree of movement: they can be *non-moveable*, such as the plates of the skull which are fused together; *slightly moveable*, such as the vertebrae of the spine; or *freely moveable*, such as the hip or shoulder.

Joint classification

Fibrous joints

Fibrous joints, sometimes referred to as fixed joints, are made up of immovable interlocking bones that are connected by tissue fibres. These fibres are mainly made up of collagen, a common tissue in the human body. A joint with bones that are able to move in some way is called an *articulated* joint, therefore a fibrous or fibro joint is a *non-articulating* joint. An example of this type of joint is the skull.

Fibrous joints need to be very strong to prevent movement of any sort, such as in the joint between the pelvis and the sacrum of the spine. This type of joint is also known as a *suture.* As there is no movement and a high degree of stability associated with this type of joint, the risk of injury is minimal and usually requires great force to do so. If injury to a fibrous joint does occur however, it is usually extremely painful and slow to heal.

Cartilaginous joints

This type of joint has slightly movable bones surrounded by ligaments that strap the joint together, as they do in other joints. Between the ends of the bones that form the joint are pads of *cartilage*, which can be compressed to allow a small degree of movement. Cartilaginous joints therefore allow a certain amount of movement, but also provide a degree of stability. The vertebral bodies and pubis symphysis (pubic bone) are examples of cartilaginous joints. As there is a certain amount of movement associated with this type of joint, the risk of injury is increased. Injury normally occurs with the cartilage discs or articular cartilage, which in most cases does not heal.

Synovial joints

Synovial joints are also referred to as freely-movable joints as they allow a great deal of movement, with the ligament straps providing most of the support. Unlike the other types, these joints contain a synovial cavity between the articulating bones that allows the range of movement mentioned above. Synovial joints also have a synovial membrane, which can secrete synovial fluid between the bones in the joint to lubricate the articulating surfaces and prevent friction. Freely moveable joints are more susceptible to injury in particular to structures such as ligaments. Some joints are more stable than others, for example, the hip joint has a deeper ball and socket so is therefore more stable than the shoulder joint, which has a shallower ball and socket. For this reason, the shoulder is more susceptible to injury.

TASK

List the three classifications of joint and briefly describe each one in relation to its structure.

Types of synovial joint

There are several types of synovial joint in the body, and they are classified according to their movement or shape. The types of synovial joint in the human body are as follows (see Chapter 3: The Muscular System for information on the movements):

Ball and socket joints

As the name suggests, this type of joint consists of a ball-like end of one bone coming together with a cup-like end of another bone (see Fig. 2.1), for example, in the shoulder and hip joint. A large degree of movement in all three

| Fig. 2.1 | **Ball and socket joint** |

Head of humerus

Scapula

planes is available in this type of joint: flexion, extension, abduction, adduction, rotation, pronation, supination, inversion, eversion and circumduction.

Hinge

In this type of joint, the convex end of one bone fits into the concave end of another bone (see Fig. 2.2). As the name suggests, the joint has a motion similar to the hinge on a door (essentially opening and closing) and examples include the elbow, knee and ankle. Only flexion and extension in one plane of movement about a single axis is possible in a joint of this kind.

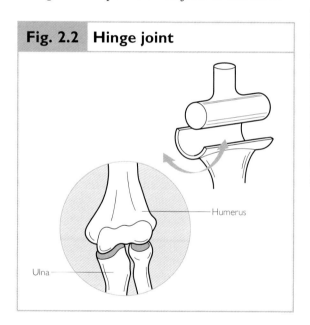

Fig. 2.2 Hinge joint

Humerus

Ulna

Gliding or plane joint

The articulating surfaces of these particular joints are usually flat or slightly curved, for example, the joints made by the carpal and tarsal bones, and the two surfaces glide over each other (see Fig. 2.3). The main movements of gliding joints are side to side and backward and forward.

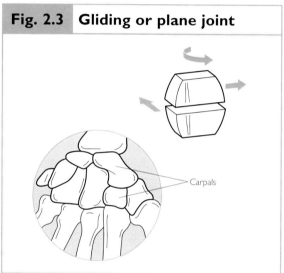

Fig. 2.3 Gliding or plane joint

Carpals

Pivot joint

In this particular joint, there is usually a rounded or pointed surface of a bone that articulates with a ring-like surface of another bone, for example the radioulnar and cervical spine (see Fig. 2.4). The movement is rotational in one axis only.

Fig. 2.4	**Pivot joint**

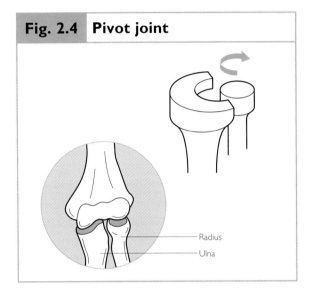

Radius
Ulna

NEED TO KNOW

The term *synovial* means 'egg-like', as synovial fluid resembles uncooked egg white.

Saddle and condyloid joint

In saddle and condyloid joints such as the thumb, concave and convex surfaces similar to a rider in a saddle fit together to allow movement in two axes, such as side to side and up and down (see Fig. 2.5). Movements include flexion, extension, abduction, adduction and circumduction.

Fig. 2.5	**Saddle and condyloid joint**

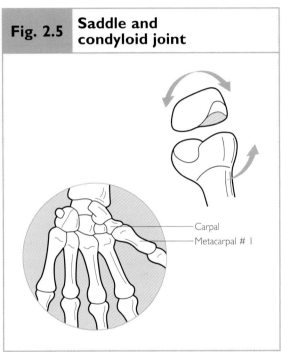

Carpal
Metacarpal # I

Typical structure of a synovial joint

All synovial joints in the body have particular characteristics in common (see Fig. 2.6):

Fig. 2.6 A typical synovial joint

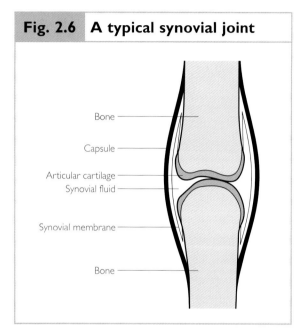

Hyaline or articular cartilage

This covers the ends of the bones that form the joint, providing smooth moving surfaces to prevent friction.

Capsular ligaments

These 'strap-like' collagen fibres hold bones together to provide support, but also to allow wanted movement.

Synovial membrane

This secretes synovial fluid, which lubricates the articular cartilage in the joint.

Joint capsule

The joint capsule consists of two layers to provide stability to the joint. The outer layer is a tough fibrous material made up of collagen and elastic fibres and is continuous with the periosteum of the articulating bones. The inner layer is the synovial membrane, which is described above.

Synovial fluid

As well as lubricating the joint surfaces, the synovial fluid contains white blood cells, which remove cellular debris, and nutrients, which nourish the articular cartilage. The synovial fluid becomes less viscous (thick) during activity, so mobilisation of the joints prior to intense activity is important.

Proprioceptors

There are many receptors in the cartilage and ligaments that provide information to the central nervous system regarding position and alignment.

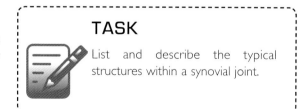

TASK

List and describe the typical structures within a synovial joint.

The effects of exercise on joints

Short-term effects

During exercise, the synovial membrane secretes synovial fluid into the joint in order to lubricate the bony surfaces and thus prevent friction. This is one of the reasons why it is important to carry out mobilisation exercises prior to the main activity, so that the joint can be lubricated before any high-impact or high-intensity exercise is undertaken.

Long-term effects

Over time, high-impact and high-intensity exercise can damage the hyaline (articular) cartilage that protects the ends of the bones. If this occurs, there may be some damage to the bone itself, resulting in a condition known as *osteoarthritis.* This can cause inflammation and pain within the joint.

Damage to ligament tissue is common as ligament has only a limited range of elasticity (up to 6 per cent). As blood supply to the ligaments is very poor, the tissues can take a very long time to heal; during the healing process the stability that the ligaments normally provide to the joint can be impaired.

The effects of pregnancy on joints

Due to the influence of the hormone relaxin, which increases in level during pregnancy, connective tissue within ligaments and tendons starts to become more elastic. This in turn will make joints less stable, particularly in the region of the pelvis and lower back. Range of movement will also increase as a result of the joint being less stable. As there is a forward shift in centre of gravity of the mother-to-be due to the uterus moving up and out of the pelvis, there tends to be an increase in lumbar lordosis (a curved lower back) which can cause considerable back pain. The pubic symphysis (bones in the pubic region) can become less stable and cause pregnancy-related pelvic girdle pain (previously known as symphysis pubis dysfunction), and in some cases separate (known as diastasis symphysis pubis) and can cause severe pelvic girdle pain. In cases such as this, almost any movements of the hips can cause discomfort or pain so it is important to try and minimise this discomfort by keeping the hips aligned and stable. Taking shorter walking strides, avoiding crossing the legs or adduction at the hip, keeping activity low-impact and short duration are all strategies that can help to minimise the pain.

EXAMPLE QUESTIONS

2.1 The tibia and the fibula make what type of joint?

a) fixed

b) cartilaginous

c) synovial

d) hinge

2.2 The facet joints of the transverse processes of the spine make what type of joint?

a) cartilaginous

b) fixed

c) synovial

d) hinge

2.3 The tibia and the femur make what type of joint?

a) fixed

b) cartilaginous

c) synovial

d) fused

2.4 The pubis symphysis is what type of joint?

a) fixed

b) cartilaginous

c) synovial

d) hinge

2.5 Which of the following is classed as a hinge joint?

a) shoulder

b) hip

c) elbow

d) wrist

EXAMPLE QUESTIONS cont.

2.6 Which two movements are available at a saddle joint?

  a) pronation and supination

  b) flexion, extension, adduction and abduction

  c) adduction and abduction only

  d) inversion and eversion

2.7 Which of the following make a joint?

  a) femur and radius

  b) ulna and tibia

  c) femur and pelvis

  d) phalanges and carpals

2.8 Which of the following make a joint?

  a) femur and ulna

  b) humerus and scapula

  c) sacrum and cervical

  d) phalanges and tarsals

2.9 Which of the following make a joint?

  a) metacarpals and phalanges

  b) fibula and radius

  c) coccyx and cervical

  d) ulna and tarsals

2.10 Which of the following make a joint?

  a) tarsals and tibia

  b) pelvis and radius

  c) sacrum and thoracic

  d) carpals and tarsals

EXAMPLE QUESTIONS cont.

2.11 Which of the following make a gliding joint?

a) bones of the spine

b) bones of the phalanges

c) bones of the carpals

d) bones of the tarsals

2.12 Which of the following make a pivot joint?

a) tibia and fibula

b) atlas and axis

c) cervical and thoracic

d) carpals and tarsals

Further reading

Abrahams, P., Craven, J. and Lumley, J. (2011) *Illustrated Clinical Anatomy* (2nd ed.), Hodder Arnold

Baechle, R.T. (2008) *Essentials of Strength Training and Conditioning* (3rd ed.), Human Kinetics

Luttgens, K. and Hamilton, N. (2008) *Kinesiology: Scientific basis of human motion* (11th ed.), McGraw-Hill

Norkin, C.C. and White, D.J. (2003) *Measurement of Joint Motion: A guide to goniometry* (3rd ed.), F.A. Davis

Porter, S. (2002) *The Anatomy Workbook*, Butterworth Heinemann

Ross, J.S. and Wilson, J.W. (2006) *Anatomy and Physiology in Health and Illness* (10th ed.), Churchill Livingstone

Sewell, D., Watkins, P. and Griffin, M. (2005) *Sport and Exercise Science: An Introduction*, Hodder Arnold

Tortora, G.J. and Grabowski, S.R. (2005) *Principles of Anatomy and Physiology* (11th ed.), Wiley

Wolfe, L. and Weissgerber, T. (2003) 'Clinical physiology of exercise in pregnancy: a literature review', *Canadian Journal of Obstetrics and Gynecology*, 25(6): 451–453

NOTES

THE MUSCULAR SYSTEM

OBJECTIVES

After completing this chapter, you will be able to:

1 Describe the differences between the three types of muscle.

2 Describe the construction of skeletal muscle.

3 Explain the process of muscle contraction and the sliding filament theory.

4 Distinguish between the properties of fast- and slow-twitch muscle fibres.

5 List and explain the types of muscle contraction.

6 Locate the major muscle groups in the body.

7 List and describe the movements available within the body.

8 Explain the different roles of muscle in the body.

9 Explain what is meant by agonist–antagonist muscle pairing.

10 List and explain the planes of movement of the body.

11 List the short- and long-term effects of exercise on muscle.

Level 2: Instructing Exercise and Fitness Knowledge

Basic Anatomy and Physiology
- The types of muscular contraction; the location and action of the major muscle groups; how voluntary muscles contract.
- Long- and short-term effects of exercise on muscles.

Level 3: Instructing Physical Activity and Exercise Knowledge

Anatomy: Muscles
- Three types of muscle (cardiac, smooth, skeletal)
  - Cardiac
    - The myocardium
    - Myocardial ischaemia – immediate impact of lack of oxygen
    - Oxygen delivery to the myocardium during exercise

- • Smooth
  - • Autonomic nervous system regulation
  - • Controlling blood pressure
- • Skeletal
  - • Structure and function of skeletal muscle (to include epimysium, perimysium, endomysium)
  - • Collagen
  - • Proprioceptors and their function (muscle spindle cells, golgi tendon organs)
  - • Muscle fibre types
- ■ Names of all major muscles and their origin and insertion
- ■ Muscle shape and actions
  - • Fibre direction and role of muscle
- ■ Muscle contraction
  - • The motor unit
  - • Axon terminals, acetylcholine, sodium ions, the action potential, the sodium–potassium pump
  - • The sliding filament theory to include sarcoplasmic reticulum, calcium ions, ATP
  - • All-or-none law of muscle physiology
  - • Muscle fatigue and oxygen debt
- ■ Types of muscle contraction (concentric, eccentric, isometric, isotonic, isokinetic)
- ■ Joint actions and muscle contraction
- ■ Agonists, antagonists, synergists and fixators applied to a range of exercises
- ■ Delayed onset muscle soreness (DOMS)
- ■ Three anatomical axes and planes
  - • Explain/label each plane and be able to describe movement in relation to the plane

Introduction

This chapter deals with the muscular system of the body, in particular the skeletal muscle system, from a perspective of structure, function and the effects of exercise. Within the National Occupational Standards framework, Level 2 and 3 instructors should be able to list the three types of muscle tissue in the human body and describe the way in which skeletal muscle contracts.

Later chapters provide physiological and biomechanical principles that, together with the anatomical knowledge covered in this chapter, provide the instructor with the understanding and ability to design appropriate exercise programmes for apparently healthy individuals and to understand the effects of various types of exercise on the human body.

Types of muscle

There are three types of muscle tissue in the body: cardiac, smooth and skeletal.

Cardiac muscle (myocardium)

The word *cardiac* refers to the heart; therefore, only the heart contains cardiac muscle. The cardiac muscle contains protein filaments called *actin* and *myosin* (see pages 40–1), as does skeletal muscle tissue, but the fibres in cardiac muscle are shorter than those in skeletal muscle. The actin and myosin protein filaments in the myocardium are arranged in disc-shaped cells that allow electrical signals to pass between the cells in order to make the heart contract.

The cardiac muscle is described as *involuntary* as no conscious thought is needed to make it contract. Contraction is initiated subconsciously by the *sinoatrial node* (SA node), which is located in the right atrium of the heart. The SA node automatically generates its own impulses that cause an electrical stimulus to spread across the heart via a network of specialist fibres. This then stimulates the ventricles to contract and pump blood into the arteries (see Chapter 7). The SA node is often known as the 'pacemaker'.

NEED TO KNOW

Pacemakers are electrical devices that are fitted to the heart to make it beat when the SA node does not function correctly. Pacemakers can automatically speed up the heart during exercise.

Due to the large number of *mitochondria* (organelles in the cardiac muscle, which use oxygen to produce energy; see Chapter 6), the myocardial cells can contract only aerobically. The cells contain large numbers of *myoglobin* (which carries oxygen) and are red in colour. The myocardium extracts a large percentage of oxygen from the blood compared to skeletal muscle. As a result, during exercise the heart has to pump more blood to supply the increased demand.

The blood flow to the heart can be reduced due to a number of reasons, for example, blockages in the blood vessels. A reduced flow of blood to the heart – known as *myocardial ischaemia* (*ische* meaning to obstruct and *emia* meaning in the blood) – leads to reduced oxygen delivery (*hypoxia*), from which the cardiac muscle cells can die. Individuals who suffer from reduced blood flow to the heart sometimes experience severe pain in the chest, neck or left arm in a condition known as *angina pectoris*, which translates as 'strangled chest'. Hypoxia can eventually lead to a heart attack (known as a *myocardial infarction* or MI) and even death. If an individual suffers from any condition that limits blood supply (*atherosclerosis*), it follows that high-intensity exercise could potentially create a problem for that individual.

NEED TO KNOW

Once cardiac muscle tissue has died it can not be regenerated by the body. Therefore, the heart becomes weaker.

Smooth muscle

Found in the walls of hollow internal structures such as the digestive system, smooth muscle automatically controls the movement of the internal systems of the body. As with other muscle tissue, smooth muscle contains actin and myosin protein filaments, but these are not as regular as they are in skeletal muscle. Smooth muscle also contracts more slowly than skeletal muscle and it maintains its contraction for longer periods. The proteins in smooth muscle are also more elastic than other muscle types.

When smooth muscle contracts, it can cause narrowing of the structures it surrounds. These include the digestive, circulatory, urinary and reproductive systems. Like cardiac muscle, smooth muscle is described as involuntary as its action is controlled by the autonomic nervous system (without conscious thought). For more on the nervous system, see Chapter 5.

NEED TO KNOW

Unlike skeletal and cardiac muscle, smooth muscle has considerable powers of regeneration.

Skeletal muscles

Skeletal muscles are normally attached from bone to bone via tendons to provide movement of the body. They are described as *voluntary* as the movement is initiated deliberately.

More than 40 per cent of the male body weight is made up of skeletal muscle tissue. The largest of this type of muscle in the body is the gluteus maximus, which is the main part of the buttock. The strongest is usually considered to be the quadricep group, even though the jaw can create a greater force. The longest is the sartorious, which runs from the iliac spine in the pelvis to the medial aspect of the tibia (top of the shin bone).

Skeletal muscles

Skeletal muscle will be covered in more detail as this will be the focus of most exercise

programmes, although cardiac muscle can also become stronger as a result of cardiovascular exercise.

Types of skeletal muscle

Skeletal muscles have many different shapes, but they can be broadly categorised into the following shape groups: parallel, pennate and convergent (see Fig. 3.1).

Parallel muscles

An example of this type of muscle is the biceps brachii in the arm, where the muscle fibres run parallel to the long axis of the muscle. In other words, the fibres run almost in a straight line from the origin to insertion. Muscles of this type are normally associated with a large range of motion.

Pennate muscles

There are two types of pennate muscle: unipennate and bipennate. Both types of muscle have a central tendon for fibre attachment that runs the length of the muscle. In a unipennate muscle the fibres attach to one side of the tendon only, whereas in a bipennate muscle the fibres attach to both sides. The fibres in all pennate muscles attach at an oblique angle and therefore have less range of motion than parallel muscles.

Convergent muscles

As the name suggests, convergent muscles have a broad origin of fibre connection that then converges to a narrow insertion. This can be seen in muscles such as the pectorals and deltoids. The range of motion in these muscles is limited, but force generation can be quite high.

Fig. 3.1	**Examples of skeletal muscle shapes**

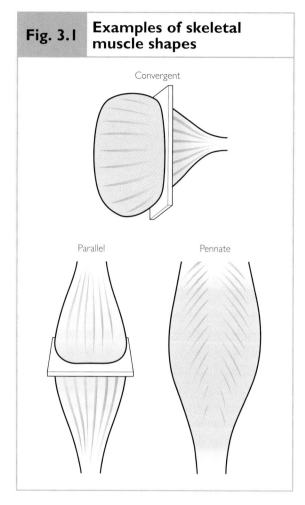

Convergent

Parallel

Pennate

TASK

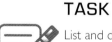

List and describe the basic functions of the three types of muscle tissue within the human body.

Structure of skeletal muscle

Skeletal muscle is mainly made up of several types of protein. The main proteins that are responsible for contraction are called *actin*

and *myosin*. Actin proteins are bound together to make thin filaments while myosin proteins are bound together to make thicker filaments. As can be seen in Fig. 3.2, the thick myosin filaments have protruding heads called *cross-bridges*. These cross-bridges 'grab hold' of the actin filaments and pull them in order to cause muscle contraction, using the chemical ATP as energy to do so (see also pages 44 and 94–5).

In the muscle, each myosin filament is surrounded by actin filaments. These protein filaments group together to form a *myofibril*, which is the smallest muscle fibre (sometimes referred to as a muscle cell). The protein filaments within a muscle fibre do not run the entire length of the muscle, but are arranged in sections called *sarcomeres*. These are the smallest units able to contract in the muscle. When the sarcomeres are laid end to end the muscles have a striped or striated appearance. This can be seen in Fig. 3.2: where the actin and myosin filaments are in rows, the muscle appears darker, but where the myosin filament has no actin filaments around it, the muscle appears lighter. Like all muscles, skeletal muscles have a good blood supply and nerve fibres to pass on the signal to contract (see Muscle contraction, pages 43–8).

Each muscle fibre is surrounded by a sheath of fibrous tissue membrane or *fascia* (meaning bandage) called *endomysium* (*endo* meaning within). This is similar to a sausage wrapped in a skin. The main protein in fascia is called *collagen*. Muscle fibres are then grouped together in a bundle (*fascicle*) and surrounded by another sheath called the *perimysium* (*peri* meaning around). Finally, another sheath called the *epimysium* (*epi* meaning upon) surrounds the entire muscle. At each end of the muscle, the three types of sheath taper off and converge to form an attachment to the bone. These attachment points are called *tendons*. See Fig. 3.3. There are also other structures within the

Fig. 3.2 Actin and myosin filaments

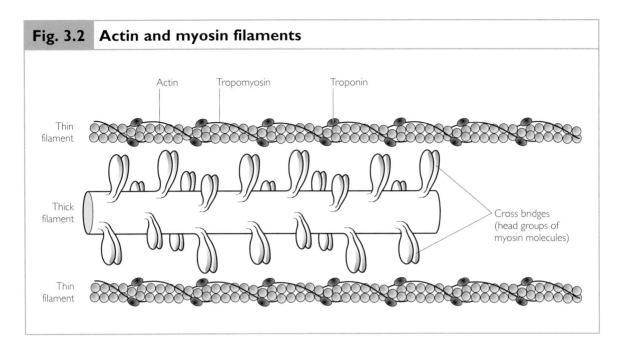

Actin — Tropomyosin — Troponin

Thin filament

Thick filament

Cross bridges (head groups of myosin molecules)

Thin filament

Fig. 3.3 A typical muscle structure

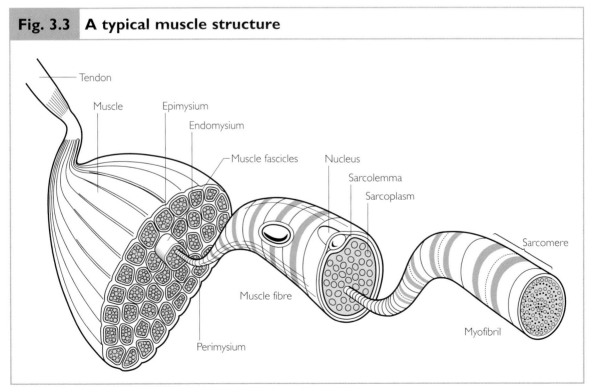

Tendon

Muscle   Epimysium

Endomysium

Muscle fascicles

Nucleus

Sarcolemma

Sarcoplasm

Sarcomere

Muscle fibre

Myofibril

Perimysium

muscle, such as *muscle spindles* and *golgi tendon organs*, which have specific roles. These two particular types of structure are known as *proprioceptors*, which refers to the way in which information regarding the position of the various body parts is relayed to the brain.

Muscle spindles

These specialist cells are sensory receptor cells located deep within the muscles. They relay information to the brain concerning the length of a muscle and the speed at which it stretches. If the muscle in which the spindle is located stretches too fast or too far, the muscle spindle causes a reflex action, making the muscle contract to prevent it becoming damaged. In other words, it causes a built-in safety device known as the *stretch reflex*. The level at which the reflex is initiated is constantly being reset by the brain.

It is also important to note that when the muscle in danger of overstretching contracts as a result of the stretch reflex, the opposing muscle (antagonist) allows it to do so by receiving a signal not to contract. This system is called *reciprocal innervation*.

Golgi tendon organs (GTO)

These are sensory receptors that lie within the tendon near its junction with a muscle. GTOs are capable of sensing tension in the tendon as a result of muscular contraction or excessive stretching. If this tension exceeds a certain threshold (set by the brain), a reflex operates that causes the muscle responsible for the tension to relax. This is known as the *tendon reflex*.

When skeletal muscles connect to bone, the attachments are known as the *origin* and *insertion*. The origin is the attachment point nearest (proximal) to the midline of the body;

NEED TO KNOW

An example of the stretch reflex is a doctor tapping their patient's knee with a small hammer. The tendon of the quadriceps is tapped, causing the muscle to stretch quickly. The stretch reflex then causes the quadriceps to contract quickly to prevent any danger.

the insertion is the attachment point furthest (distal) from the midline. Every muscle has its own nerve supply and is stimulated to contract by the brain sending an electrical impulse or *twitch*. All muscles are in a state of readiness to contract or respond to a signal from the brain. This state of tension has been described as *tone*. By exercising on a regular basis, the amount of muscle tone in the body can be increased, as can the size of a muscle; this is known as *hypertrophy* (*hyper* meaning excessive and *trophy* meaning nourishment). The opposite of this, muscle shrinkage, is known as *atrophy*.

Following a period of strenuous exercise it is common for skeletal muscles to become sore. This soreness, associated with post-exercise self-perception, has been termed *delayed onset muscle soreness* (DOMS). Even though the exact mechanism of this soreness is not fully understood, scientists have found that following periods of intense exercise there is considerable damage at a microscopic level, which may be related to DOMS.

NEED TO KNOW

The gastrocnemius muscle in the lower leg can contain over 1,000,000 fibres.

Muscle contraction

The main function of skeletal muscle is to provide movement for the body through contraction. When a muscle contracts, the protein filaments within the muscle fibre slide over one another with the aid of small projections or cross-bridges. This is known as the *sliding filament* theory (see Fig. 3.6).

Several steps occur before the proteins actually move over each other to cause muscle contraction:

1. The brain sends an electrical signal (or 'action potential') to the muscle fibre via a pathway or nerve known as a *motor neuron* (see Fig. 3.4). The motor neuron has long branches called *axons* down which the electrical signals can travel. Each motor neuron can make connections with many muscle fibres, depending on the role of the muscle: in the small muscles of the eye, the motor neuron might make connection with only a few muscle fibres, whereas in the quadriceps a motor neuron might make contact with thousands of muscle fibres. A motor neuron and the fibres it stimulates to contract are called a *motor unit*. If an action potential is sent, all of the fibres in the motor unit will contract, known as the *all or none* principle. It is not possible to make only some of the fibres fed by the motor unit signal contract.

2. At the end of each motor neuron axon, in close proximity to the muscle fibre to be contracted, is an *axon terminal*. The axon terminal physically spreads out to become larger than the axon itself. This part is called the *synaptic end bulb* because it looks like a bulb and is next to a gap or *synapse*. When the action potential reaches the synaptic end bulb, it causes depolarisation of the covering of the end bulb (the *presynaptic*

Fig. 3.4   A typical motor neuron

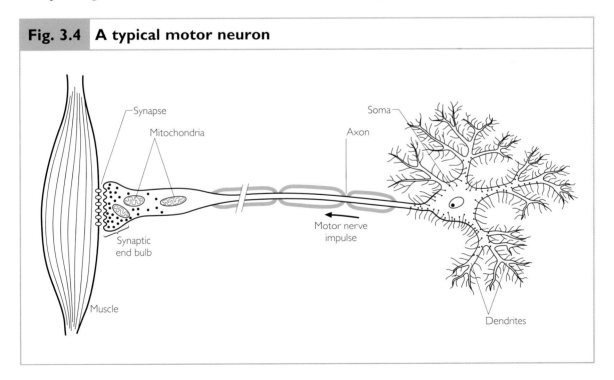

membrane). Depolarisation is a process in which the movement of sodium and potassium ions (charged particles) causes an electrical current to flow. This is regulated by something known as the *sodium–potassium pump*. The depolarisation process enables a neurotransmitter called *acetylcholine* (Ach), which is stored in the end bulb, to be released across the gap between the presynaptic membrane of the end bulb and the *postsynaptic membrane* (where Ach is collected by the muscle) of the muscle fibre (see Fig. 3.5). The motor neuron axon and the muscle fibres do not physically touch.

3. When enough acetylcholine reaches the postsynaptic membrane of the muscle fibre it can depolarise the membrane. This creates an action potential that stimulates the release of calcium from its store in the *sarcoplasmic reticulum*, which surrounds each myofibril. The calcium uncovers 'binding sites' on the actin molecules that provide a connection for the cross-bridges on the myosin molecules. The cross-bridges are like arms that pull the actin and myosin protein molecules across each other (see also pages 40–1).

4. *Adenosine triphosphate* (ATP) is the fuel within the body that provides the energy for the cross-bridges to pull the actin and myosin proteins (muscle fibres) together. This action is known as muscle contraction.

Each electrical signal (twitch) lasts for a very short time, so the brain needs to keep sending the signals to maintain the muscle contraction. When the brain stops sending the signals, the muscle returns to its original length.

TASK

Briefly describe how muscle contracts as if you were explaining it to someone with no knowledge of physiology.

Types of muscle fibre

Even though there are many different types of muscle fibre, they are usually grouped into two types: fast- and slow-twitch. The term 'twitch' refers to the brief contraction of all the muscle fibres in a motor unit in response to a single electrical impulse from the brain. In slow-twitch fibres each contraction lasts for between 100 and 200 milliseconds, whereas in fast-twitch fibres the contraction lasts for under 100 milliseconds. The two broad categories of fibre differ with respect to the speed and force of the contraction and the type of fuel they use to do this.

Slow-twitch (type I) muscle fibres

Slow-twitch fibres, otherwise known as slow-oxidative or SO, are the smallest type of fibres and are used for endurance-type activities and posture control. They have many mitochondria (see page 96) and therefore use oxygen and

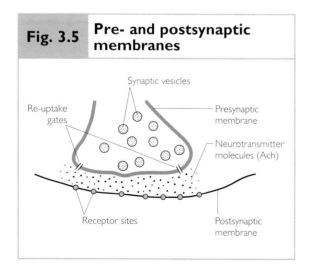

Fig. 3.5 Pre- and postsynaptic membranes

Synaptic vesicles

Re-uptake gates

Presynaptic membrane

Neurotransmitter molecules (Ach)

Receptor sites

Postsynaptic membrane

Fig. 3.6 The 'sliding filament' theory

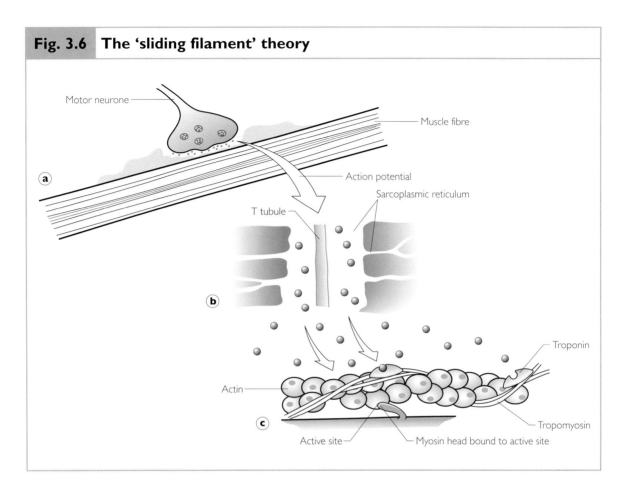

Motor neurone

Muscle fibre

Action potential

Sarcoplasmic reticulum

T tubule

Troponin

Actin

Tropomyosin

Active site

Myosin head bound to active site

a **b** **c**

fat as their main fuel source for contraction. The number and size of mitochondria can be increased by endurance training, which means that more oxygen can be delivered to the muscle for the same intensity of exercise, leading to a greater energy output.

Slow-twitch fibres also have many capillaries to supply blood. These fibres are good at extracting oxygen from the blood as they contain large amounts of myoglobin, which is the oxygen carrier in the muscle. The myoglobin also gives the fibres a reddish colour. As can be seen in Fig. 3.7, slow-twitch fibres contract smoothly and do not generate as much force as fast-twitch fibres, but are more resistant to fatigue.

Fast-twitch (type II) muscle fibres

Fast-twitch (type II) fibres are powerful, but are quick to fatigue. Generally, they have fewer mitochondria, and therefore use glucose as their main fuel source. As the amount of myoglobin is less, they appear white in colour.

Fast-twitch fibres can be split into two groups: type IIa and type IIb.

Type IIa fibres

Type IIa fibres are also known as fast oxidative glycolytic (FOG) fibres because they can use both oxygen (aerobic) and glucose (anaerobic) as a fuel to contract. Like slow-twitch fibres, type

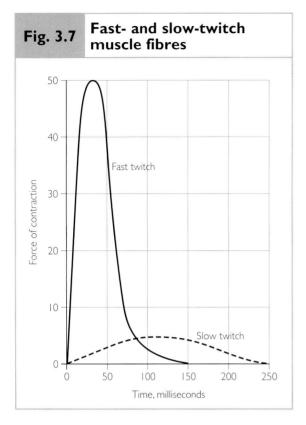

Fig. 3.7 **Fast- and slow-twitch muscle fibres**

fuel to contract. They are the most forceful and largest of the muscle fibres and are used when type I and type IIa fibres can't cope with the workload of an exercise. Type IIb fibres have limited amounts of mitochondria and myoglobin and therefore look white in comparison to slow-twitch fibres. These fibres can generate more force than other types, because the space left due to the lack of mitochondria is filled with more contractile proteins such as actin and myosin. Because the fibres are solely anaerobic, however, they are quick to fatigue compared to slow-twitch fibres.

Table 3.1 shows the common characteristics of the three groups of muscle fibres.

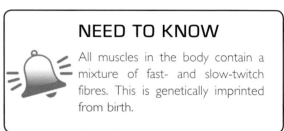

NEED TO KNOW

All muscles in the body contain a mixture of fast- and slow-twitch fibres. This is genetically imprinted from birth.

IIa fibres contain large amounts of capillaries and myoglobin that allows them to contract aerobically, but also contain stores of glycogen so that they can contract anaerobically. Type IIa fibres can produce more force than type I fibres, but not as much as type IIb fibres. Similarly, the contraction speed and force generation of these fibres is greater than type I fibres but not as great as type IIb fibres. Type IIa fibres are also known as intermediate fibres because they are between Ia and IIb fibres in terms of size. Type IIa fibres are used when type I fibres can't cope with the workload of an exercise.

Type IIb fibres

Type IIb fibres are also known as fast glycolytic (FG) fibres as they can only use glucose as a

Fibre distribution and modification

Most skeletal muscles contain a mixture of all three types of muscle fibre, but their proportion varies depending on the usual action of the muscle. For example, postural muscles have a higher proportion of type I fibres as they are normally required to contract for long periods of time and therefore need to be resistant to fatigue. Muscles such as those of the shoulders and arms, which are not constantly active but are used intermittently to produce large amounts of tension, such as in lifting and throwing, have a higher proportion of type IIa and type IIb fibres.

Even though most skeletal muscles are a mixture of all three types of fibre, the muscle fibres in any one motor unit are all the same. In addition, the different muscle fibres within a

Table 3.1	Common characteristics of muscle fibre types		
	Type I	Type IIa	Type IIb
Contraction time	Slow	Fast	Very fast
Size of motor neuron	Small	Large	Very large
Resistance to fatigue	High	Intermediate	Low
Activity used for	Aerobic	Long-term anaerobic	Short-term anaerobic
Force production	Low	High	Very high
Mitochondrial density	High	High	Low
Capillary density	High	Intermediate	Low
Oxidative capacity	High	High	Low
Glycolytic capacity	Low	High	High
Major storage fuel	Triglycerides	CP, glycogen	CP, glycogen

muscle may be used in various ways, depending on need. For example, if only a weak contraction is needed in a certain muscle to perform a task, only type I fibres are activated by their motor units in that muscle. If a stronger contraction is needed, the motor units of type IIa fibres are activated in conjunction with those of type I fibres in that muscle. If a maximal contraction is required, all motor units within that muscle are activated. Motor unit recruitment always follows the same order of smaller type I motor units followed by type IIa then type IIb larger motor units as can be seen in Fig. 3.8.

Although the number of each type of muscle fibre within a particular muscle never changes, the characteristics of those present can be altered through exercise. Endurance-type exercises, such as running or swimming, result in cardiovascular and respiratory changes that mean the skeletal muscles receive better

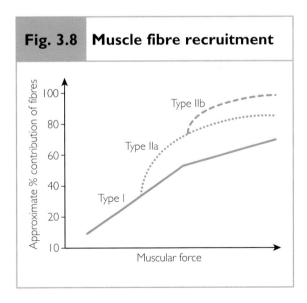

Fig. 3.8 Muscle fibre recruitment

supplies of oxygen and carbohydrates. This causes a gradual adaptation in the characteristics of type IIb fibres into the characteristics of type IIa fibres. The transformed muscle fibres show a slight increase in diameter, mitochondria, blood capillaries and strength. These changes do not contribute to increased muscle mass. On the other hand, exercises that require great strength for short periods of time, such as weightlifting, produce an increase in the size and strength of type IIb fibres. However, we are what we were born with and can influence the characteristics of our muscle fibres only by a small percentage.

TASK

List and describe the common characteristics of the different types of skeletal muscle fibres.

Types of muscle contraction

Muscle contractions are classified according to what happens to the length of the muscle in the contraction.

Isotonic contractions

Isotonic contractions occur when a muscle contracts while lifting and lowering a resistance against gravity. This type of contraction can be divided into two types: *concentric* and *eccentric*. A type of contraction known as *isokinetic* (meaning same speed) is normally used only with specialised testing equipment.

Concentric contractions

A concentric contraction occurs when the muscle doing the work (the *prime mover* or *agonist*) shortens in length when contracting against a resistance. In other words, the ends of

the muscle come together, for example, in the lifting stage of a bicep curl when the weight is being lifted upward. When using free weights, the muscle doing the main work is always contracting concentrically when the weight is moving upward, against gravity. This is slightly different with resistance machines (the system of pulleys means that the limb moving the weight may not be moving upward against gravity, but the weights stack will be), but the muscle doing the main work will be working concentrically when the weight stack is moving up.

Eccentric contractions

An eccentric contraction occurs when the muscle acting as the prime mover gets longer when contracting against a resistance, for example, when the weight is being lowered during a bicep curl. Here, the ends of the muscle are moving away from each other. In fast movements, muscles working eccentrically have a braking effect.

Isometric contractions

An isometric contraction occurs when there is no change in muscle length when contracting against a resistance, for example, if a weight is lifted and then held still so that the ends of the muscle do not move either together or away from each other. From a programme design point of view, it is important to be aware that isometric contractions can raise blood pressure.

TASK

Briefly describe the terms eccentric, concentric and isometric.

The roles of muscle in the body

The role of an individual muscle can change depending on the type of exercise or activity it is participating in at a specific time. These roles are normally categorised into the following groups: *agonists*, *antagonists*, *synergists* and *stabilisers*. Table 3.2 describes each role.

Agonist–antagonist pairs

Muscles are said to work in pairs across joints as they can only pull (contract) and not push. Imagine a muscle pair such as the biceps brachii and triceps brachii in the arm. When the bicep contracts with greater force, it decreases the angle of the joint (flexion), while the tricep stretches to allow this movement. In contrast, when the tricep contracts with greater force than the bicep, it increases the angle of the joint (extension) and the bicep stretches to allow the movement. If both muscles contracted with the same amount of force or tension, the joint angle would not move.

The muscle that contracts with the most force is called the agonist and causes the joint to move. The other muscle of the pair is called the antagonist. The amount of force produced by the antagonist can vary. Take the example of kicking a ball. The quadriceps muscles are the agonist group as they contract to extend the knee joint. The hamstrings are the antagonist group as they try to control the speed of the extension by contracting slightly. This is known as co-contraction. The amount of co-contraction in the antagonist muscle will decrease through practice of the movement.

When strength training, it is important that both agonists and antagonists are trained to create muscle balance. If either the agonist or antagonist is much stronger or less flexible than the other, the joint that is crossed by the two muscles may be pulled out of alignment to create poor posture. For example, if the quadriceps are much stronger than the hamstrings, they will pull on the point of attachment at the front of the pelvis (the rectus femoris) and tilt the pelvis forward. In turn, this will lead to an increase in the curvature of the lumbar spine, known as hyperlordosis (see page 19). This is the case for muscle pairs at all joints: there are published guidelines as

Table 3.2	Roles of different muscle types
Type I	Description
Agonist	A muscle that is responsible for the main action or movement (also known as the prime mover). For example, the agonist in a shoulder press is the deltoid muscle group.
Antagonist	A muscle that directly opposes the agonist. For example, the antagonist in a shoulder press is the latissimus dorsi.
Fixator	A muscle that stabilises a joint so the other muscles (agonists) are able to move the levers around the joint. For example, the transversus abdominis is a stabiliser for the pelvis.
Synergist	A muscle that helps the agonist to carry out its movement. For example, the tricep is a synergist for the bench press.

to typical strength ratios between the pairs (for example, Norkin and White, 1995) that should be reflected in any strength training programme.

Planes of movement

Planes are a useful way of describing movements of the body. The term *plane* is used to describe an imaginary flat surface at various angles to the body. Movement of the human body can occur in three planes: *sagittal*, *frontal* and *transverse* (see Fig. 3.9).

Sagittal (or median) plane

The sagittal or median plane splits the body into left and right sides (but not necessarily equal halves). The movements distinctive to this plane are flexion and extension. Examples of resistance exercises in this plane include bicep curls, leg extensions, front deltoid raises and tricep push downs.

Frontal (or coronal) plane

The frontal or coronal plane divides the body into front and back sections. The movements distinctive to this plane are abduction and adduction. Examples of resistance exercises in this plane include lateral pull-downs, shoulder press and lateral shoulder raises.

Transverse (or horizontal) plane

The transverse or horizontal plane splits the body into upper (superior) and lower (inferior) sections. The movements distinctive to this plane are medial (internal) and lateral (external) rotation. An example of a resistance exercise in this plane is a chest press.

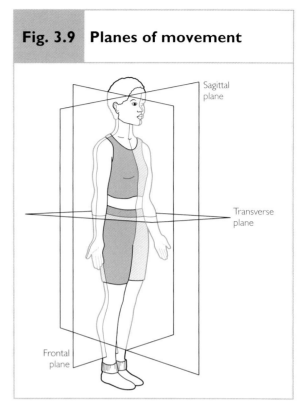

Fig. 3.9 Planes of movement

Sagittal plane

Transverse plane

Frontal plane

Exercises or movements can place various amounts of stress on joints depending on which plane of movement is used to perform the exercise. For example, the ligaments in the knee joint allow it to move in the sagittal plane, but are stressed in the frontal and transverse planes. For rehabilitation purposes, exercises are often prescribed in relation to the plane of movement for a particular joint.

TASK

Choose five resistance training exercises. Name the agonist, antagonist, synergists and stabilisers for each exercise and state the plane in which the movement occurs.

Muscle and movement

As a health and fitness instructor it is useful to know the names and locations (including origins and insertions) of the major muscle groups in the body (see Fig. 3.10 (a) and 3.10 (b)) and the movements they create when contracting. When muscles contract, they either create movement or stabilise the bones that they are attached to. There are many terms used in anatomy to describe movements of the body. It can help to remember some of these movements by linking them to specific resistance training exercises. Common terms and associated exercises are listed from page 52.

Fig. 3.10	Figure 3.10 (a) Major muscle groups (front view) (b) Major muscle groups (rear view)

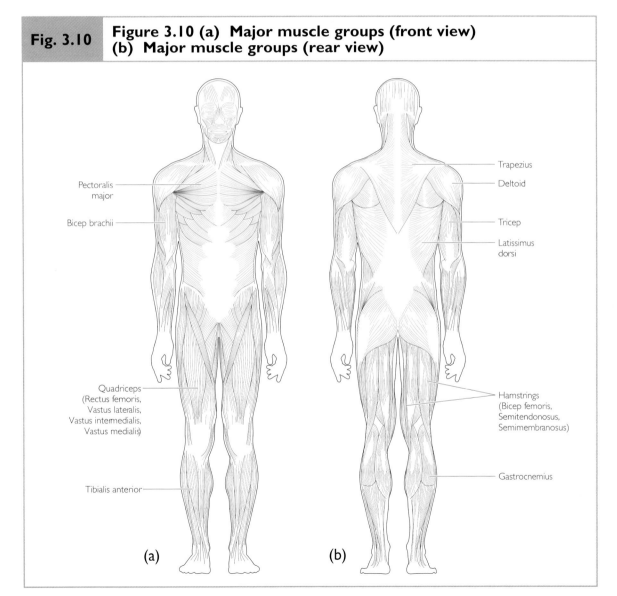

(a)

(b)

Pectoralis major

Bicep brachii

Quadriceps (Rectus femoris, Vastus lateralis, Vastus intermedialis, Vastus medialis)

Tibialis anterior

Trapezius

Deltoid

Tricep

Latissimus dorsi

Hamstrings (Bicep femoris, Semitendonosus, Semimembranosus)

Gastrocnemius

Flexion

The term flexion (*flex-* meaning to bend) is used when the angle between the moving bones gets smaller, for example, the forearm coming toward the upper arm in a Bicep Curl. Another example is illustrated in Fig. 3.11, where the torso is bent forward. This is known as forward flexion of the spine or trunk.

Fig. 3.11	Forward flexion of the trunk

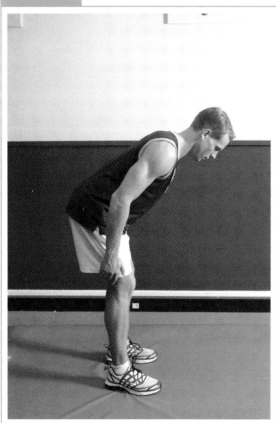

Extension

Extension (*exten-* meaning to stretch) is the opposite of flexion and occurs when the joint angle gets larger. An example of this is a straight-leg movement in a backward direction in the sagittal plane, such as a Hip Extension. Another example is shown in Fig. 3.12, where the torso is bent backward from a flexed position. This is known as extension of the spine or trunk.

Fig. 3.12	Extension of the trunk

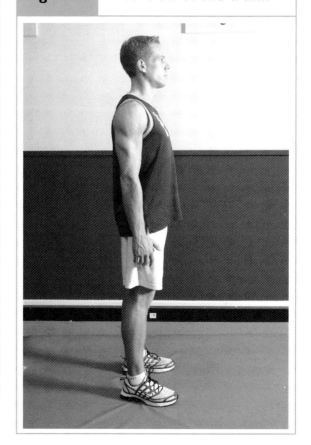

Hyperflexion/extension

The word hyper (meaning more than or excessive) in this sense refers to a movement beyond the normal range of motion for a particular joint.

Lateral flexion/extension

This refers to bending to the side. An example is shown in Fig. 3.13, known as lateral flexion or extension of the spine or trunk.

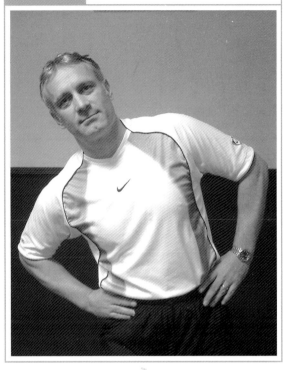

Fig. 3.13 **Lateral flexion/ extension of the trunk**

Abduction

Ab- means away and *-duct* means to lead, and the term abduction is used to describe a movement away from the midline of the body (see Fig. 3.14a). An example is a Lateral Shoulder Raise, where the arm moves away from the body in the frontal plane. Horizontal abduction is a term used to describe the limb moving away from the body in a horizontal motion such as the humerus motion in a seated row.

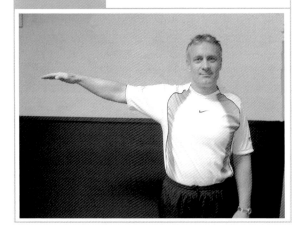

Fig. 3.14a Abduction

Adduction

Ad- means toward, and the term adduction is used to describe a movement toward the midline of the body (see Fig. 3.14b). An example of this is a Lat Pull-down. Horizontal adduction is a term used to describe the limb moving towards the body in a horizontal motion such as the humerus motion in a chest press.

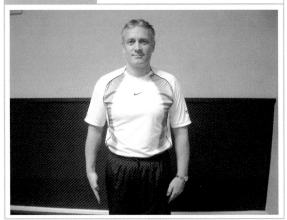

Fig. 3.14b Adduction

Rotation

This term is used to describe a bone revolving around its own axis, for example, rotation at the ulna–radius joint when turning the palm face down from a face-up position and vice versa (see Fig. 3.15). Another example is the head rotating from side to side, as if saying no.

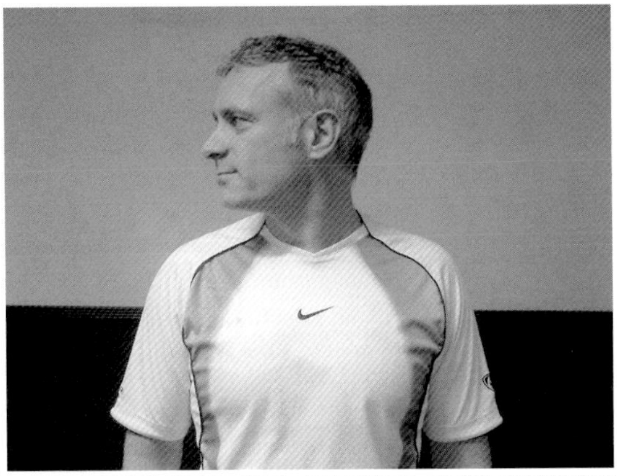

Fig. 3.15b **Rotation**

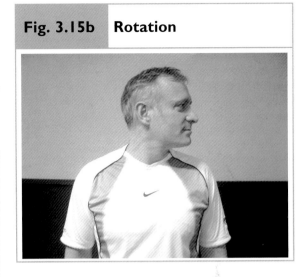

Fig. 3.15a **Rotation**

Medial rotation

This term describes any inward rotational movement, for example, when the upper arm (humerus) rotates toward the body (see Fig. 3.16a). This is a common resistance exercise used for the muscles known as the Shoulder 'Rotator Cuff'.

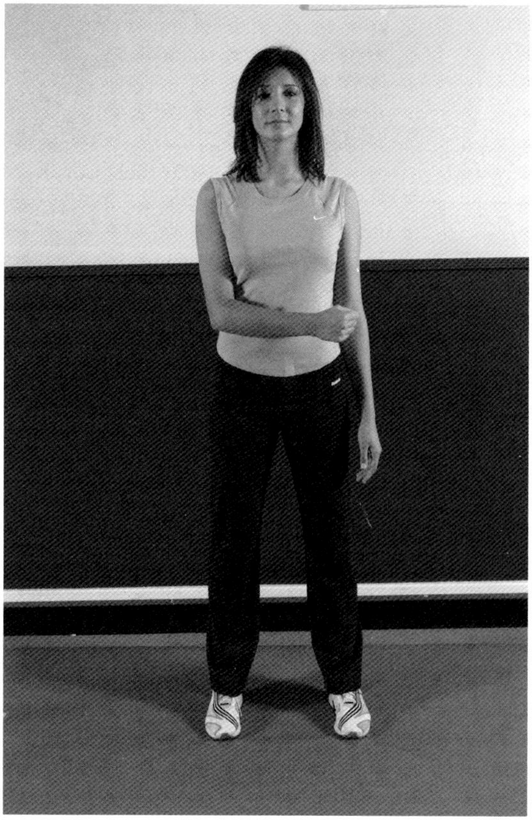

Lateral rotation

This term describes any outward rotational movement, for example, when the upper arm (humerus) rotates away from the body (see Fig. 3.16b). This is also a Rotator Cuff exercise.

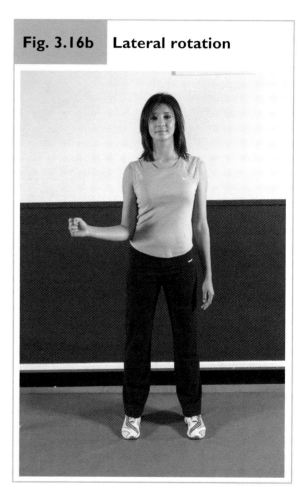

Fig. 3.16a   **Medial rotation**

Fig. 3.16b   **Lateral rotation**

Elevation and depression

Elevation describes an upward movement of a part of the body, such as lifting the shoulders up in a shoulder shrug exercise. Depression refers to a downward movement of a part of the body, such as the shoulders going down from an elevated position. See Figs 3.17a and b.

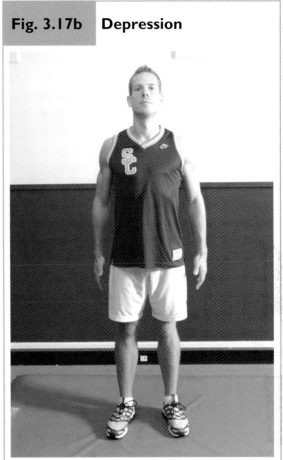

Fig. 3.17b **Depression**

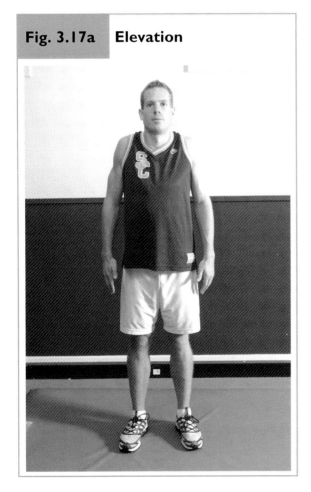

Fig. 3.17a **Elevation**

Retraction and protraction

Retraction refers to a movement that involves drawing part of the body back, for example pulling the shoulders back from a protracted position. Protraction describes a movement that involves part of the body going forward in the transverse plane. For example, when the shoulders go forward, this is known as protraction. See Figs 3.18a and b.

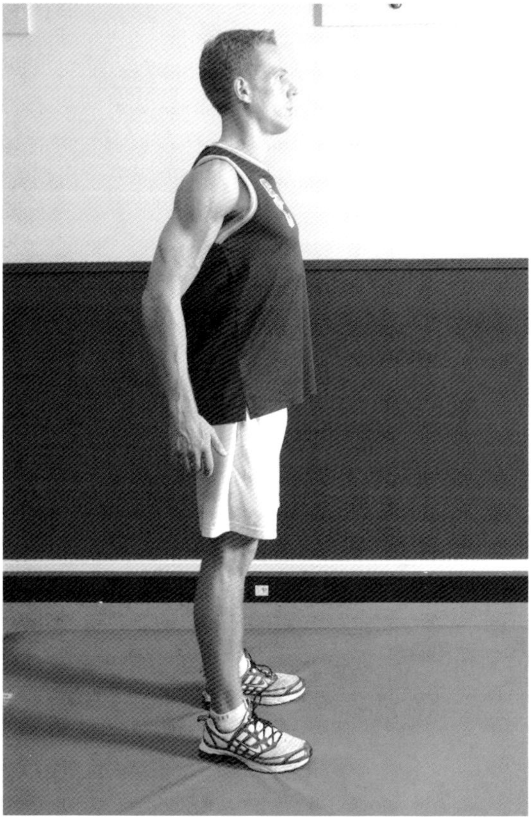

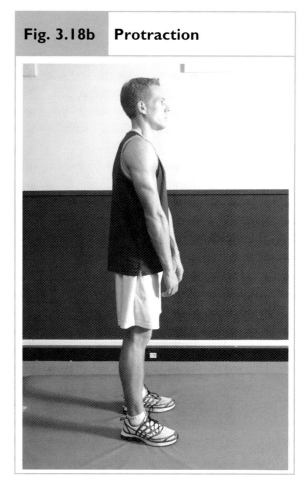

Fig. 3.18b   Protraction

Fig. 3.18a   Retraction

Pronation and supination

Pronation is used to describe the palm of the head or the sole of the foot being turned down; supination is used to describe the palm of the hand or the sole of the foot being turned up. See Figs. 3.19a and b.

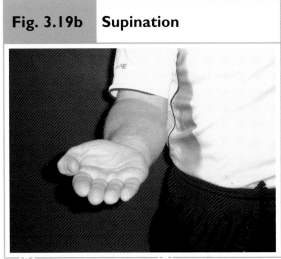

Fig. 3.19b   Supination

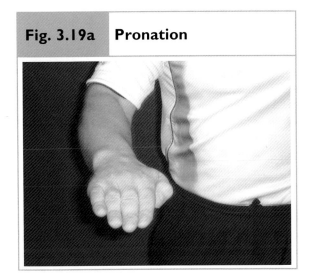

Fig. 3.19a   Pronation

Inversion, eversion, plantar flexion and dorsiflexion

Inversion occurs when the sole of the foot is turned inward, while eversion describes the foot being turned outward. Plantar flexion refers to bending the foot at the ankle joint so the foot is pointing down, while dorsiflexion refers to bending the foot at the ankle joint so the foot is pointing up. See Figs 3.20a–d.

Fig. 3.20	(a) Inversion; (b) Eversion; (c) Plantar flexion; (d) Dorsiflexion

Major muscles: their location and available movement

Individual muscles can be responsible for several movements depending on the position of the associated limbs. The following tables provide an overview of the locations and main movements of the major muscles.

Table 3.3 Locations of the muscles of the shoulder joint/girdle

	Origin	Insertion
Pectoralis major	Clavicle and sternum	Proximal part of humerus
Pectoralis minor	External surfaces of 3rd-5th ribs.	Coracoid process of scapula.
Serratus anterior	Outer surfaces of upper 8 or 9 ribs.	Anterior surface of medial border and inferior angle of scapula.
Trapezius	Base of skull (occipital bone). Spinous processes of cervical 7 and all thoracic vertebrae.	Lateral 3rd of clavicle. Acromion process. Spine of scapula.
Rhomboid major/minor	Spinous processes of 7th cervical and upper 5 thoracic vertebrae.	Medial border of scapula.
Latissimus dorsi	Illiac crest, sacrum, lumbar and lower thoracic vertebrae	Proximal anterior part of humerus
Deltoid	Distal 1/3rd of clavicle (anterior fibres) and whole ridge of scapula (posterior fibres)	Lateral mid-part of humerus
Biceps brachii (also elbow flexion)	Top of the scapula	Proximal part of radius
Triceps brachii (also elbow extension)	Long head – scapula Lateral head – humerus Medial head – humerus	Olecranon of ulna Olecranon of ulna Olecranon of ulna
Supraspinatus	Groove in top of scapula	Lateral head of humerus
Subscapularis	Underneath of scapula	Medial head of humerus
Infraspinatus	Flat body of scapula	Lateral/posterior head humerus
Teres minor	Lateral medial wing of scapula	Posterior head of humerus
Teres major	Lateral inferior wing of scapula	Medial proximal 1/3rd of humerus
Levator scapulae	Transverse processes of first 3 or 4 cervical vertebrae.	Upper medial border of scapula.

Table 3.4 Movements of the muscles of the shoulder joint/girdle

	Shoulder flexion	Shoulder extension	Shoulder abduction	Shoulder adduction	Medial rotation	Lateral rotation	Protraction	Retraction	Elevation	Depression
Pectoralis major				x	x					
Pectoralis minor							x			x
Serratus anterior							x			
Trapezius								x*m*	x*u*	x*l*
Rhomboid major/minor								x		
Latissimus dorsi		x		x	x					
Deltoid	x*f*	x*p*	x		x*f*	x*p*				
Biceps brachii	x									
Triceps brachii		x								
Supraspinatus			x							
Subscapularis					x					
Infraspinatus				x		x				
Teres minor		x		x		x				
Teres major		x		x*a*	x*a*					
Levator scapulae								x*a*	x	

Key: *p* = posterior fibres, *f* = anterior fibres, *u* = upper fibres, *m* = middle fibres, *l* = lower fibres, *a* = assists

Table 3.5	Locations of the muscles of the hip joint	
	Origin	Insertion
Hip flexors: Rectus femoris Iliopsoas (Iliacus/psoas major)	Bottom front of pelvis. Last thoracic and lumbar. vertebrae and front of the pelvis.	Proximal anterior part of tibia. Proximal medial part of femur.
Hip extensors: Gluteus maximus	Sacrum, coccyx and medial posterior of pelvis (Iliac crest).	Proximal posterior third of femur.
Hamstrings: Biceps femoris Semimembranosus Semitendinosus	Ischium for all and bicep femoris has attachment to the femur.	Head of the fibula and lateral side of tibia for biceps femoris. Proximal lateral posterior part of tibia for other two.
Hip adductors: Adductor brevis Adductor longus Adductor magnus Gracilis Pectineus	Pubic bone for all and Ischium as well for adductor magnus.	Proximal third posterior femur. Posterior middle part of femur. Whole posterior of femur. Proximal inside part of tibia. Proximal medial part of femur.
Hip abductors: Gluteus medius Gluteus minimus Tensor fascia latae Piriformis Sartorius Tensor fascia latae	Posterior middle part of pelvis for minimus and medius lies above this (Ilium). Posterior lateral part of pelvis for TFL. Front of sacrum for piriformis. Anterior superior iliac spine for sartorius.	Proximal lateral part of femur (greater trochanter) for min and med. Proximal lateral side of tibia for TFL. Top of greater trochanter for piriformis. Upper medial surface of tibia for sartorius.

Table 3.6	Movements of the muscles of the hip joint					
	Hip flexion	Hip extension	Hip abduction	Hip adduction	Hip lateral rotation	Hip medial rotation
Rectus femoris	×					
Iliopsoas	×				×	
Biceps femoris		×				
Semimembranosus		×				
Semitendinosus		×				
Adductor brevis	×			×		×
Adductor longus	×			×		×
Adductor magnus	×f	×p		×		×
Gracilis				×		×
Pectineus	×			×		
Sartorius	×		×		×	
Gluteus maximus		×			×	
Gluteus medius			×			×
Gluteus minimus			×			×
Tensor fascia latae	×		×			
Piriformis			×hf		×	

Key: f = anterior fibres, p = posterior fibres, hf = when in hip flexion

Table 3.7	Locations of the muscles of the knee and ankle joints	
	Origin	Insertion
Quadriceps: Vastus lateralis Vastus medialis Vastus intermedius Rectus femoris	Whole of femur, lateral, medial and anterior for all vastus (and greater trochanter for lateralis). For rectus femoris see the hip joint (page 63)	Proximal anterior part of tibia (via patella into tibial tuberosity).
Hamstrings: Bicep femoris Semitendonosus Semimembranosus	See hip joint (page 63)	See hip joint (page 63)
Calf: Gastrocnemius Soleus	Distal medial and lateral femur (condyles) for gastroc. Proximal fibula and medial tibia for soleus.	Calcaneus (through Achilles tendon) for both.
Tibialis anterior	Proximal lateral half of the tibia.	First metatarsal in the foot.

Table 3.8	Movements of the muscles of the knee and ankle joints				
	Knee flexion	Knee extension	Plantarflexion	Dorsiflexion	Inversion
Vastus lateralis		×			
Vastus medialis		×			
Vastus intermedius		×			
Rectus femoris		×			
Bicep femoris	×				
Semitendonosus	×				
Semimembranosus	×				
Gastrocnemius	×		×		
Soleus			×		
Tibialis anterior				×	×

Table 3.9	Locations of the muscles of the trunk	
	Origin	Insertion
Rectus abdominis	Pubis and Pubic Symphysis.	Xiphoid process of sternum and costal cartilage of 5, 6, 7th ribs.
Erector spinae: (Iliocostalis, longissimus, spinalis)	Slips of muscle arising from sacrum, Iliac crest, spinous and transverse processes, ribs.	Ribs, spinous and transverse processes. Occipital bone.
Multifidus	Posterior surface of sacrum and processes of vertebrae.	Spinous processes 2–4 vertebrae superior of origin.
Quadratus lumborum	Iliac crest and Iliolumbar ligament.	12th rib and transverse processes of upper 4 lumbar vertebrae.
Transversus abdominis	Cartilage of lower ribs, inguinal ligament, anterior iliac crest, thoracolumbar fascia.	Pubis and linea alba.
Diaphragm	Xiphoid process. Lower six ribs and their cartilage. Upper 2 or 3 lumbar vertebrae.	All fibres converge to a central tendon.
Internal obliques	Iliac crest, inguinal ligament and thoracolumbar fascia.	Cartilage of last 4 ribs and linea alba.
External obliques	Xiphoid process of sternum and costal cartilage of 5, 6, 7th ribs.	Anterior portion of the iliac crest and linea alba.
Pelvic floor: (levator ani and the coccygeus muscles)	Inner surface of the pelvis and ischium.	Sacrum and coccyx.

TASK

Try to identify all of the major muscles in the body and list their origins, insertions and main movements.

Effects of exercise on muscle

Short-term effects

The short-term effects of exercise on muscle include the following:

1. Capillary dilation, which allows for increased blood supply.
2. Increased muscle temperature, which increases pliability (stretch) and power.
3. Increased oxygen demand and usage by muscles being used in order to supply the increased number of fibres being used.
4. Muscle fibres contract at a faster rate due to increased nerve stimulation. The contracting muscle fibres, which squeeze the walls of blood vessels, push blood further along the vessels in a type of pump action known as the 'muscle pump'.

Long-term effects

The long-term effects of exercise on muscle include the following:

1. Improved muscle tone.
2. Improved posture.
3. Increase in muscle bulk (hypertrophy) and strength. This is due to an increase in the number of contractile proteins (actin and myosin), an increase in the number and size of myofibrils per muscle fibre, and increased amounts of connective, tendinous and ligamentous tissues.
4. Increased numbers of enzymes and stored nutrients.
5. Increased number of capillaries and mitochondria in slow-twitch fibres.

EXAMPLE QUESTIONS

3.1 What is the main fuel of type I fibres?
a) fat and oxygen
b) protein
c) glucose
d) creatine phosphate

3.2 What is the main fuel of type IIb fibres?
a) fat and oxygen
b) protein
c) glucose
d) alcohol

3.3 Which type of muscle can be found in the digestive system?
a) striated
b) cardiac
c) skeletal
d) smooth

3.4 Which type of muscle can be found in the heart?
a) striated
b) cardiac
c) skeletal
d) smooth

3.5 In muscle contraction, which hormone is released from the end motor plate and crosses the synaptic gap?
a) adenosine triphosphate
b) acetyl choline
c) actin
d) myosin

EXAMPLE QUESTIONS cont.

3.6 Which term is used to describe a muscle under tension where the origin and insertion move away from each other?

a) isometric
b) concentric
c) eccentric
d) isokinetic

3.7 Which term is used to describe a muscle under tension where the origin and insertion move closer together?

a) isometric
b) concentric
c) eccentric
d) isokinetic

3.8 What is the name given to a muscle when performing the role of stabilising a joint?

a) agonist
b) antagonist
c) synergist
d) fixator

3.9 What is the name given to a muscle when performing the role of assisting the agonist muscle?

a) agonist
b) antagonist
c) synergist
d) fixator

3.10 What is the name given to a muscle when performing the main action?

a) agonist
b) antagonist
c) synergist
d) fixator

EXAMPLE QUESTIONS cont.

3.11 Which exercise is associated with the sagittal plane?
a) lateral raise
b) hip abduction
c) pull down
d) leg extension

3.12 Which exercise is associated with the frontal or coronal plane?
a) chest press
b) hip extension
c) pull down
d) leg extension

Further reading

Abrahams, P., Craven, J. and Lumley, J. (2011) *Illustrated Clinical Anatomy* (2nd ed.), Hodder Arnold

Alter, M.J. (2004) *Science of Flexibility* (3rd ed.), Human Kinetics

Baechle, R.T. (2008) *Essentials of Strength Training and Conditioning* (3rd ed.), Human Kinetics

Benjamin, H.J. and Glow, K.M. (2003) 'Strength training for children and adolescents', *Physical Sports Medicine*, 31: 19–27

Fry, A.C. (2004) 'The role of resistance exercise intensity on muscle fibre adaptations', *Sports Medicine*, 34: 663–679

Kraemer, W.J., and Ratamess, N.A. (2006) 'Hormonal responses and adaptations to resistance exercise and training', *Sports Medicine*, 35: 339–361

Marieb, E.N. (2009) *Human Anatomy and Physiology* (8th ed.), Benjamin Cummings

Norkin, C.C. and White, D.J. (2003) *Measurement of Joint Motion: A guide to goniometry* (3rd ed.), F.A. Davis

Porter, S. (2002) *The Anatomy Workbook*, Butterworth Heinemann

Ross, J.S. and Wilson, J.W. (2006) *Anatomy and Physiology in Health and Illness* (10th ed.), Churchill Livingstone

Sewell, D., Watkins, P. and Griffin, M. (2005) *Sport and Exercise Science: An Introduction*, Hodder Arnold

Tortora, G.J. and Grabowski, S.R. (2005) *Principles of Anatomy and Physiology* (11th ed.), Wiley

NOTES

CARTILAGE, LIGAMENTS AND TENDONS

4

OBJECTIVES

After completing this chapter, you will be able to:

1 Describe the structure and function of cartilage.

2 List and describe the different types of cartilage and give examples of each.

3 Describe the structure and function of ligaments.

4 List and describe the common ligaments found in joints of the body.

5 Describe the structure and function of tendons.

6 List the short- and long-term effects of exercise on cartilage, ligaments and tendons.

Level 3: Instructing Physical Activity and Exercise Knowledge

Anatomy

- Articulations and joint movements.

- Structure and movement potential/anatomical limitations of major joints (shoulder, hip, knee, elbow).

- Muscle attachment sites.

- Stability vs movement within each type of joint.

- Ligaments; articular cartilage.

Introduction

This chapter deals with connective tissue within the human body, in particular cartilage, ligament and tendon, from a perspective of structure, function and the effects of exercise. Within the National Occupational Standards framework, Level 2 and 3 instructors should be able to list the types and roles of cartilage and ligament in the human body.

Later chapters provide physiological and biomechanical principles that, together with the anatomical knowledge covered in this chapter, provide the instructor with the understanding and ability to design appropriate exercise programmes for apparently healthy individuals and to understand the effects of various types of exercise on the human body.

Cartilage

Structure, function and types

Cartilage is a dense, tough connective tissue that forms only a very small portion of the adult skeleton. It consists of a mixture of collagen (*colla* meaning glue) and elastic fibres and has similar properties to plastic, in that it can withstand compression but can tear with combined twisting and compression movements. Cartilage has hardly any blood supply (known as *avascular*), so when it becomes damaged it cannot really repair itself. If it does, the process is slow and not always complete.

There are three types of cartilage in the body: *hyaline* or *articular*, *fibro* and *elastic*. As far as health and fitness instructors are concerned, only articular and fibro cartilage is important as they can both be affected by exercise, while elastic cartilage cannot.

Hyaline or articular cartilage

Hyaline or articular cartilage is a thin, tough, shiny, smooth bluey-white membrane. It covers the ends of bones that form cartilaginous (slightly moveable) and synovial (freely moveable) joints, and its function is to prevent friction between the opposing surfaces in joints. This occurs when the cartilage becomes lubricated with synovial fluid, which is secreted by a synovial membrane (see page 30). Moving a joint through its range of movements before an exercise session begins is called mobilisation, and stimulates the release of synovial fluid to prevent friction in the joint during exercise.

Fibro cartilage

Fibro cartilage is thick, strong and spongy and acts as a shock absorber in joints such as the spine (intervertebral bodies) and the knee (menisci). This type of cartilage is mainly made up of collagen.

Elastic cartilage

Elastic cartilage is made up of bundles of elastic fibres that provide flexible support. Examples are found in the ear and nose.

Ligaments

Structure and function

Ligaments are tough, white, non-elastic fibrous tissues strung together in a strap-like formation. They are attached from bone to bone and allow wanted movement while preventing unwanted movement. Ligaments have poor blood supply, so their healing time is slow. Depending on the severity of the damage to the ligament, it can take weeks to months for the healing process to be complete. However, ligaments can become stronger and in some cases hypertrophy (become larger) following weight-bearing activities.

Common ligaments in the body

Many ligament structures can be found throughout the body, acting as straps or bindings for specific joints. The following provides an overview of the main ligaments and their function in relation to specific movements at the associated joint. Ligaments allow certain movement to take place at the joint, and for the purpose of this book it is assumed that the ligaments prevent all other movements at the joint.

Ligaments of the knee

The *medial* and *lateral collateral* ligaments are located on the medial and lateral aspects of the

Fig. 4.1	**Common ligaments of the knee**

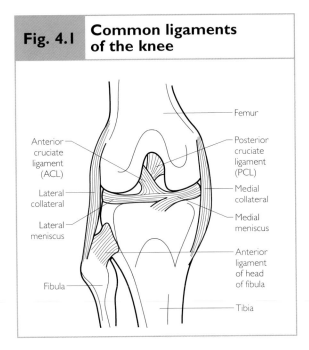

Fig. 4.2	**Common ligaments of the shoulder**

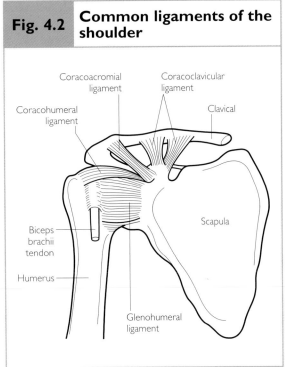

knee joint, and allow knee flexion and extension while preventing any other movement. The *anterior* and *posterior cruciate* ligaments are located within the knee joint between the femur and tibia and prevent the two bones from sliding away from each other. See Fig. 4.1.

Ligaments of the shoulder

The main ligaments in the shoulder joint are the:

- Coracohumeral ligament
- Glenohumeral (superior, middle and inferior) ligaments
- Coracoacromial ligament.

As the shoulder joint is a freely moveable synovial joint, it requires a certain degree of movement in all directions. The ligament structures in the joint allow this movement, but provide stability at the end ranges and prevent the humerus from pulling out of the glenoid cavity (known as a luxation). See Fig. 4.2.

Ligaments of the ankle

The ligaments of the ankle can be separated into medial and lateral groups, and the names of the ligaments are taken from the bones to which they attach so they can easily be identified.

The *medial* ligaments are a group of ligaments called the *deltoids*, which comprise the following:

- Calcaneotibial – between the calcaneous and the tibia
- Anterior and posterior talotibial – between the talus and the tibia
- Tibionavicular – between the tibia and the navicular.

The *lateral* ligaments, known as the *lateral collateral* ligaments, are made up of the following:

- Calcaneofibular – between the calcaneus and the fibula
- Anterior and posterior talofibular – between the talus and the fibula.

Between them, the deltoid and lateral collateral ligaments allow the foot to move in flexion and extension, but provide stability in lateral movements such as inversion and eversion. In other words, they prevent the ankle from rolling in or out. See Fig. 4.3.

Ligaments of the pelvis

The ligaments of the pelvis are required to support a fibrous joint and therefore need to be as strong as possible to prevent any movement whatsoever. The main ligaments of the pelvic girdle are:

- Sacroiliac – between the sacrum and ilium
- Sacrosciatic – between the iliac crest and ischium

There are no muscle attachments across the sacroiliac or pubic joints and so they are dependent on ligaments for stability. Cartilage lines the surfaces of the joints and a pad of cartilage between the pubic bones, at the symphysis pubis, acts as support, shock absorption and to maintain stability and alignment of the pelvis. See Fig 4.4.

Ligaments of the hip

The main ligaments of the hip are:

- Ischiofemoral – between the ischium and the femur
- Iliofemoral – between the ilium and the femur
- Pubofemoral – between the pubis and the femur

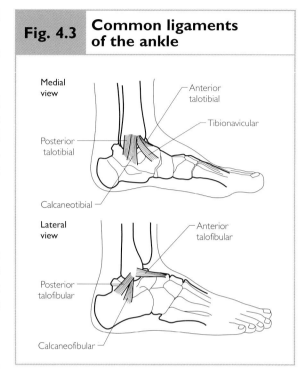

Fig. 4.3 Common ligaments of the ankle

Medial view
Anterior talotibial
Tibionavicular
Posterior talotibial
Calcaneotibial

Lateral view
Anterior talofibular
Posterior talofibular
Calcaneofibular

As the hip joint is classed as a freely-moveable synovial joint, it requires a certain degree of movement in all directions. The ligament structures in the hip joint allow this degree of movement but also provide a certain amount of stability at the end ranges and prevent the femur from pulling out of its socket called the acetabulum (this is known as a luxation). See Fig 4.5.

Fig. 4.4 | Common ligaments of the pelvis

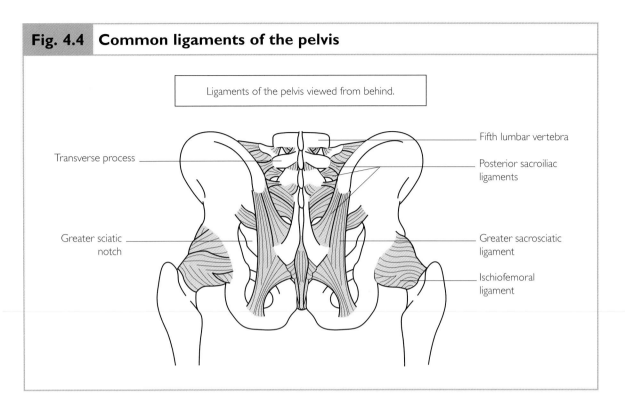

Ligaments of the pelvis viewed from behind.

Transverse process

Greater sciatic notch

Fifth lumbar vertebra

Posterior sacroiliac ligaments

Greater sacrosciatic ligament

Ischiofemoral ligament

Fig. 4.5 | Common ligaments of the hip

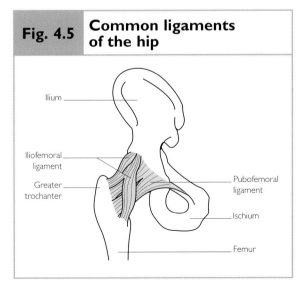

Ilium

Iliofemoral ligament

Greater trochanter

Pubofemoral ligament

Ischium

Femur

Tendons

Structure and function

Tendons are bluish-white, slightly elastic fascia tissues that connect muscles to bone. Tendons are made up of the sheaths that surround the muscle fibres and attach to the periosteum covering on the bone. In some cases the area of connection is relatively small, for example, the biceps brachii tendons, but in other cases the tendon can be spread out in sheets over a wide area, such as the tibialis anterior. The latter type of tendon attachments are called *aponeuroses.*

When muscles contract they pull from the middle and therefore exert a pulling force on the tendons at each end of the muscle. As the tendons are connected to bone, they will attempt to pull the bones together. If one of the bones remains in a fixed position, the other bone will move towards it and create movement.

Tendons stretch only slightly and not as much as muscle tissue, and prolonged tension on tendon tissue may result in tearing. Tendons are reasonably slow to heal as their blood supply is less than that of muscles. As with ligaments, tendons will become stronger with weight-bearing activity.

In the case of extreme force, it is also possible for the tendon to pull away from the attachment point at the periosteum. This is called an *avulsion*. This can be a partial tear, where there is still some tendon attached, or a complete rupture, where the entire tendon is torn from the periosteum. If a complete rupture occurs, the muscle will have no attachment at one end and will therefore be unable to move the bone it is attached to. This requires surgery, whereas a partial tear can heal in time. Tendons can also become inflamed through repetitive use. This type of injury is known as tendonitis (*itis* meaning inflammation).

The effects of exercise on cartilage, ligament and tendon

Short-term effects

During exercise, there will be an increased blood supply to both ligaments and tendons. As a result, heat will be produced, which makes these structures slightly more elastic and less susceptible to injury. Also during exercise, synovial fluid is released from synovial membranes in the joints, which lubricates articular cartilage.

Long-term effects

Both ligaments and tendons are capable of becoming stronger after a long-term period of regular exercise, in particular resistance training. Ligaments can actually hypertrophy (grow in size) by a small amount. An excessive amount of exercise has been linked to damage of both fibrous and articular cartilage.

TASK

Describe the structure and function of cartilage (all types), ligament and tendon tissue.

EXAMPLE QUESTIONS

4.1 What type of cartilage can be described as a thin, tough, shiny, bluey-white membrane?

  a) fibro

  b) elastic

  c) articular

  d) tendonous

4.2 What type of cartilage can be described as bundles of fibres that provide flexible support?

  a) fibro

  b) elastic

  c) articular

  d) tendonous

4.3 What type of cartilage can be described as a thick, strong and spongy shock-absorber?

  a) fibro

  b) elastic

  c) articular

  d) tendonous

4.4 What is fibro cartilage mainly made up of?

  a) elastin

  b) collagen

  c) tendon

  d) fascia

4.5 Which is a ligament of the knee?

  a) coracohumeral

  b) calcaneotibial

  c) lateral collateral

  d) ischiofemoral

EXAMPLE QUESTIONS cont.

4.6 Which is a ligament of the shoulder?

a) lateral collateral

b) calcaneotibial

c) coracohumeral

d) Ischiofemoral

4.7 Which is a ligament of the hip?

a) ischiofemoral

b) calcaneotibial

c) lateral collateral

d) coracohumeral

4.8 Which is a ligament of the ankle?

a) coracohumeral

b) calcaneotibial

c) lateral collateral

d) ischiofemoral

4.9 Which type of tissue connects bone to bone?

a) cartilage

b) tendon

c) ligament

d) muscle

4.10 Which type of tissue connects muscle to bone?

a) cartilage

b) tendon

c) ligament

d) muscle

EXAMPLE QUESTIONS cont.

4.11 What is the name of the fibro cartilage in the knee joint?
   a) collateral
   b) periosteum
   c) intervertebral
   d) meniscus

4.12 Which type of tissue does the statement 'allows wanted but prevents unwanted movement' relate to?
   a) cartilage
   b) tendon
   c) ligament
   d) muscle

Further reading

Abrahams, P., Craven, J. and Lumley, J. (2011) *Illustrated Clinical Anatomy* (2nd ed.), Hodder Arnold

Baechle, R.T. (2008) *Essentials of Strength Training and Conditioning* (3rd ed.), Human Kinetics

Porter, S. (2002) *The Anatomy Workbook*, Butterworth Heinemann

Ross, J.S. and Wilson, J.W. (2006) *Anatomy and Physiology in Health and Illness* (10th ed.), Churchill Livingstone

Sewell, D., Watkins, P. and Griffin, M. (2005) *Sport and Exercise Science: An Introduction*, Hodder Arnold

Tortora, G.J. and Grabowski, S.R. (2005) *Principles of Anatomy and Physiology* (11th ed.), Wiley

NOTES

THE NERVOUS AND
ENDOCRINE SYSTEMS

5

OBJECTIVES

After completing this chapter, you will be able to:

1 Describe the structure and function of the nervous system.

2 Describe the structure and function of the endocrine system.

3 Describe the roles of sensory receptors in the body.

4 Explain the roles of the autonomic and somatic branches of the peripheral nervous system.

5 Explain the roles of the sympathetic and parasympathetic branches of the autonomic nervous system.

6 List the glands and associated hormones of the endocrine system.

7 Describe the role of hormones within the endocrine system.

Level 3: Instructing Physical Activity and Exercise Knowledge

Anatomy: Nervous and endocrine systems

■ Role of the nervous system:

• Sensory input
• Interpretation
• Major output

■ Two parts of the nervous system:

• Central (CNS)
• Peripheral (PNS) – autonomic and somatic

■ How regular activity can enhance neuromuscular connections and improve motor fitness

■ Endocrine glands and associated hormones involved in exercise preparation and performance:

• Pancreas – regulation of blood glucose
• Adrenal glands – adrenalin

■ Testosterone

Introduction

This chapter deals with the nervous and endocrine systems within the human body from a perspective of structure, function and the effects of exercise. Within the National Occupational Standards framework, Level 2 and 3 instructors should be able to explain and describe how both systems work within the human body.

Later chapters provide physiological and biomechanical principles that, together with the anatomical knowledge covered in this chapter, provide the instructor with the understanding and ability to design appropriate exercise programmes for apparently healthy individuals and to understand the effects of various types of exercise on the human body.

Overview of the nervous and endocrine systems

Although the nervous system and the endocrine system are separate, they work in conjunction with each other to monitor and regulate all of the systems within the body, including temperature, blood pressure, blood glucose and blood calcium. When the nervous and the endocrine systems work optimally to keep all of the other systems within limits, the body is said to be in *homeostasis*.

The main difference between the two systems is in the way they operate. The nervous system operates as a network of connecting nerve fibres that rapidly transmit electrical signals, whereas the endocrine system operates more slowly using chemical messengers called *hormones* that are secreted into the bloodstream from groups of cells known as *glands*. It is worth noting that when these hormone messengers are released from nerve endings as opposed to glands, they are known as *neurotransmitters*.

Both the nervous and the endocrine systems work on a 'lock and key' basis: the messengers (neurotransmitters and gland hormones) act as keys, and the places they deliver messages to are called locks (or *receptor cells*). Messages will only be accepted by locks if they are the correct keys: in other words, specific neurotransmitters and hormones can deliver messages only to specific sites. If the specific key is not available, there will be no effect on the lock. Take, for example, beta-blockers (commonly prescribed medication for heart conditions). If beta receptor cells combine with beta keys, the resulting message stimulates an increase in heart rate. In the case of cardiac patients, where limiting the heart rate is a necessity, chemicals that block the beta receptor cells, and thus prevent an increase in heart rate, are prescribed. These are called beta-blockers for obvious reasons.

NEED TO KNOW

It was once thought that nerve damage could never be repaired, but scientists have had recent success with regeneration of nerve tissue.

The nervous system

The nervous system has many functions in the body, for example, being responsible for our perceptions, memories and behaviour, as well as being responsible for muscle contraction.

Structure of the nervous system

The nervous system is divided into two parts: the central nervous system (CNS) and the peripheral nervous system (PNS). The CNS is made up of the brain, brainstem and the spinal cord (see Fig. 5.1).

The PNS is made up of a series of nerve branches that either lead into or away from the CNS. Nerves that lead away from the CNS are called *motor* or *efferent* nerves, as they carry information to muscles and organs to affect a response. Nerves that lead into the CNS are called *sensory* or *afferent* nerves as they carry information back to the CNS about changes in the body.

Nerves that lead into the CNS come from groups of specialised cells around the body called *sensory receptors*. As the name implies, sensory receptors are capable of detecting changes in the body such as temperature, sight, hearing, taste and smell. Table 5.1 lists some receptors and their functions in the body.

TASK

List the common sensory receptors in the human body and give a brief description of what each one does.

When the body is in homeostasis, the sensory receptors do not relay information to the brain. If any changes are detected by the receptors away from homeostasis, information is then relayed to the brain via the sensory or afferent nerves so the brain can initiate a response. For example, if proprioceptors in the ankle ligaments detect that they are being stretched too far, the brain will respond by sending electrical twitches via the motor or efferent nerves to specific leg muscles in order to balance and stabilise the ankle.

Table 5.1	Description of sensory receptors
Receptor	Description
Proprioceptors	These are found in tissue such as muscle, tendon and joints and provide information relating to position. These receptors can be damaged easily in injuries such as ankle sprains. If this occurs, balance can be affected because of a lack of position information being relayed to the brain.
Baroreceptors	This type of receptor is mainly found in the walls of blood vessels in order to relay information to the brain regarding blood pressure.
Chemoreceptors	These receptors monitor the concentration of certain chemicals in the body, such as blood glucose level.
Thermoreceptors	These are present in all tissues of the body to detect changes in temperature.
Nociceptors	These are present in all tissues of the body and detect pain (tissue damage).

Fig. 5.1	The central nervous system (CNS)

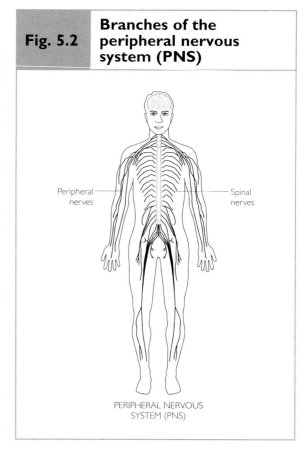

CENTRAL NERVOUS
SYSTEM (CNS)

Fig. 5.2	Branches of the peripheral nervous system (PNS)

PERIPHERAL NERVOUS
SYSTEM (PNS)

Branches of the peripheral nervous system

The peripheral nervous system has two branches, known as the *somatic branch* and the *autonomic branch*. The autonomic branch is then further subdivided into two branches, called the *sympathetic* and *parasympathetic* branches (see Fig. 5.2).

In simple terms, the somatic nervous system controls voluntary actions such as moving away from danger or foul smells, while the autonomic nervous system controls involuntary actions such as heart rate and blood pressure.

Sympathetic nervous system

This branch of the nervous system acts almost like a stimulus to increase specific activity or stimulate specific processes in the body. Sympathetic nerves do this by releasing the neurotransmitters *adrenaline* and *noradrenaline* (as discussed on page 84, these are hormones but are called neurotransmitters as they are not secreted from glands). These neurotransmitters speed up processes in the body. For instance, adrenaline stimulates the breakdown of fat and glycogen to be used for energy production.

Parasympathetic nervous system

This branch of the nervous system has the opposite effect to that of the sympathetic nervous system: its main roles are reducing the activity of processes within the body and conserving fuel stores. The main neurotransmitter used in this system is acetylcholine (Ach), which is used in the process of muscle contraction (see pages 43–8).

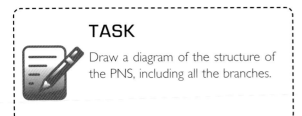

TASK

Draw a diagram of the structure of the PNS, including all the branches.

The endocrine system

As discussed above, the nervous system sends messages (information) around the body by using neurotransmitters, which are hormones secreted by nerve endings. The endocrine system is another messenger system for the body that sends messages using hormones secreted by glands. This is normally done in conjunction with the nervous system: if the homeostasis of the body is disturbed, the nervous system recognises this and in turn stimulates specific glands in the body to release hormones, which try to return the body to homeostasis. Most hormones are circulated via the bloodstream, so the endocrine system can be quite slow compared to the nervous system.

The main endocrine glands include the pineal, pituitary, thyroid, parathyroid and adrenal glands (see Fig. 5.3). The pineal and pituitary glands are located in the brain, whereas the other glands and tissues are located around the body. There are other tissues in the body that secrete hormones, such as the hypothalamus, pancreas, thymus, ovaries, testes, kidneys and stomach, but these are not referred to as endocrine glands. Table 5.2 provides an overview of the common glands and tissues and their function related to the release of hormone messengers in the body.

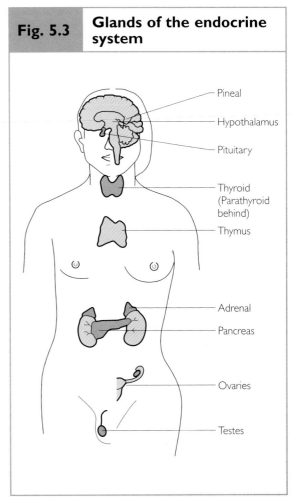

Fig. 5.3 **Glands of the endocrine system**

NEED TO KNOW

Seasonal Affective Disorder (SAD), which is mainly related to the hormone melatonin, affects about 25 per cent of the population.

Types of hormones

There are two main groups of hormones: lipid-soluble and water-soluble.

Lipid-soluble hormones

One common type of lipid-soluble hormone is *steroid* hormones. Cortisol, testosterone and oestrogen (among others) belong to this group. Steroid hormones take a reasonable amount of time to have an effect, but their effect is usually long lasting. The main functions of this group are related to either growth function or the control of cycles in the body such as the menstruation cycle.

Water-soluble hormones

One common type of water-soluble hormones is *peptide* hormones. Examples include insulin and glucagon, which are used to control blood sugar levels. The main role of this group of hormones is to act on metabolism.

TASK

List the common glands and tissues in the body and the hormones that they secrete.

Table 5.2	Roles of the common glands and tissues
Gland/tissue	**Role**
Pituitary	Produces mainly trophic hormones that stimulate other glands and also growth hormone which stimulates growth and cell reproduction.
Pineal	Releases melatonin to promote sleep.
Thyroid	Tyrosine based hormones that regulate metabolism.
Parathyroid	Produces hormones that control bone growth by regulating calcium levels in the body.
Adrenal glands	Produces hormones such as adrenalin, cortisol, aldesterone and noradrenaline (catecholamines and corticosteroids are group names) which are responsible for the increase in nutrient breakdown and also stress response.
Pancreas	Responsible for the production of insulin and glucagon into the bloodstream in order to control blood sugar levels.
Testes and ovaries	Produces sex hormones such as testosterone and estrogen to regulate reproductive function.

EXAMPLE QUESTIONS

5.1 Glands are responsible for secreting what into the bloodstream?
a) glucose
b) neurotransmitters
c) hormones
d) ATP

5.2 Nerve endings are responsible for secreting what?
a) neurotransmitters
b) ATP
c) hormones
d) glucose

5.3 Nerves that lead away from the central nervous system are known as what?
a) motor or afferent
b) motor or efferent
b) sensory or efferent
d) sensory or afferent

5.4 Nerves that lead back to the central nervous system are known as what?
a) sensory or afferent
b) sensory or efferent
c) motor or efferent
d) motor or afferent

5.5 Which of the following receptors sense position?
a) proprioceptors
b) chemoreceptors
c) nociceptors
d) thermoreceptors

EXAMPLE QUESTIONS cont.

5.6 Which of the following receptors sense pain?

a) proprioceptors

b) chemoreceptors

c) nociceptors

d) thermoreceptors

5.7 Which of the following receptors sense temperature?

a) proprioceptors

b) chemoreceptors

c) nociceptors

d) thermoreceptors

5.8 Which of the following receptors sense chemical composition?

a) proprioceptors

b) chemoreceptors

c) nociceptors

d) thermoreceptors

5.9 Catecholamines and corticosteroids are secreted by which gland?

a) pituitary

b) parathyroid

c) pancreas

d) adrenals

5.10 Tyrosine based hormones that regulate metabolism are secreted by which gland?

a) pituitary

b) thyroid

c) pancreas

d) adrenals

EXAMPLE QUESTIONS cont.

5.11 Glucagon is secreted by which gland?

a) pituitary

b) parathyroid

c) pancreas

d) adrenals

5.12 Testosterone and oestrogen are secreted by which gland?

a) pituitary

b) parathyroid

c) pancreas

d) testes and ovaries

Further reading

Abrahams, P., Craven, J. and Lumley, J. (2011) *Illustrated Clinical Anatomy* (2nd ed.), Hodder Arnold

Baechle, R.T. (2008) *Essentials of Strength Training and Conditioning* (3rd ed.), Human Kinetics

Porter, S. (2002) *The Anatomy Workbook*, Butterworth Heinemann

Ross, J.S. and Wilson, J.W. (2006) *Anatomy and Physiology in Health and Illness* (10th ed.), Churchill Livingstone

Sewell, D., Watkins, P. and Griffin, M. (2005) *Sport and Exercise Science: An Introduction*, Hodder Arnold

Tortora, G.J. and Grabowski, S.R. (2005) *Principles of Anatomy and Physiology* (11th ed.), Wiley

NOTES

ENERGY SYSTEMS

6

OBJECTIVES

After completing this chapter, you will be able to:

1 Name and describe the structure of ATP used for muscle contraction.
2 Name and describe each system within the body that can produce ATP.
3 Explain how each energy-producing system is contributing at low, medium and high exercise intensities.
4 Name the by-products of each energy-producing system.
5 Explain the problems associated with lactic acid.
6 Suggest ways to prevent depletion of glucose stores in the body.
7 Name typical activities associated with each energy-producing system as the main contributing system.
8 Explain how fitness levels can affect the energy-producing systems being used.

Level 2: Instructing Exercise and Fitness Knowledge

Basic Anatomy and Physiology
- The aerobic and anaerobic energy systems and the energy requirements of physical activity.

Level 3: Instructing Physical Activity and Exercise Knowledge

Energy Systems
- ATP
- Three energy systems:
  - CP, anaerobic, aerobic
  - Interaction of the energy systems during a range of exercises/activities
  - Capacity of the three energy systems and adaptations in relation to training modalities
  - Effects of exercise intensity, duration and fitness levels on the energy systems used
- Use of energy nutrients at different intensities and amount of energy nutrients used at different intensities

Introduction

This chapter deals with the supply of fuel to the muscles of the body, known as *energy systems*, and in particular the interaction of the various systems during rest and during different intensities of exercise. Within the National Occupational Standards framework, Level 2 and 3 instructors should be able to describe each of the different systems as well as describe how these interact during rest and exercise.

This chapter provides the instructor with the understanding of how energy systems work, which will provide the underpinning knowledge to assist in the design of appropriate exercise programmes for apparently healthy individuals and in understanding the effects of various types of exercise on the human body.

Energy systems for muscular contraction

Whether the body is at rest or moving during exercise, energy must be supplied either to living systems for chemical reactions to take place or to the muscles for movement to occur. The unit of energy that is used in the body for muscles to contract is called *adenosine triphosphate* (ATP), which is sometimes known as the *energy currency* in the body.

An ATP molecule is made up of the adenosine part (a molecule of adenine and a molecule of ribose) with three (*tri* meaning three) phosphate groups bonded to each other (see Fig. 6.1).

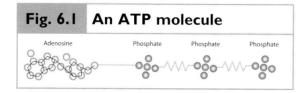

Fig. 6.1   An ATP molecule

The bonds keeping the phosphates together are known as *high-energy bonds*. If one of the phosphates is split from the adenosine molecule, a large amount of energy is released to be used for muscle contraction (see Fig. 6.2). Heat is also given off when a phosphate splits from the adenosine. This leaves an adenosine molecule with only two phosphates, which is called *adenosine diphosphate* or *ADP* (*di* meaning two).

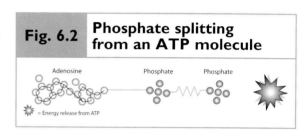

Fig. 6.2   Phosphate splitting from an ATP molecule

The main problem with this is that there is only enough ATP in the body to last for about four seconds, so a phosphate must be re-attached to the ADP to make ATP in order for the process to start again. This is called *re-synthesis*. Carbohydrates, fats and proteins are digested to provide a source of phosphate.

This process of re-synthesis occurs on a continuous basis in the body, but the amount of energy in the form of ATP that is needed depends on the amount of muscle contraction or exercise being carried out: obviously, when exercising at a higher level, more ATP is needed to supply the energy. The place in the muscle where the ATP is used to provide energy for muscle contraction is called the *mitochondria* (see also page 38) or the 'powerhouse'.

Carbohydrates are used to supply energy in the form of ATP mainly in the short term, and fats are used mainly in the long term. Protein is usually used only as a standby source of ATP energy. There are three systems within the body that supply the energy from the digested food to the muscles that need it: the creatine phosphate (ATP–CP) system, the *aerobic* system and the *anaerobic* system.

The creatine phosphate system (ATP–CP)

This system is also known as the PCr or Phosphocreatine system. As ATP stores last only for a few seconds, the body needs a system that can re-synthesise ADP to ATP very quickly when an individual starts to exercise. The creatine phosphate system can do this almost immediately, but the body contains only a very short-term supply. As a result, the system can be used for up to about 10 seconds only, but can be used over and over again as long as a recovery period of about three minutes is allowed (this recovery period can be low-intensity exercise). Once the creatine phosphate molecule has given its phosphate to the ADP, which in turn becomes ATP, a phosphate can be broken off to release energy (see Fig. 6.3).

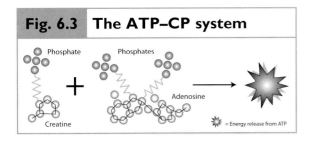

| Fig. 6.3 | **The ATP–CP system** |

This system is very simple and produces no waste products. However, it is not very efficient: for every one molecule of creatine phosphate used, only one molecule of ATP is produced. After the store of creatine phosphate in the body has been used, the body must switch to another system to supply phosphate in order to re-synthesise ADP. Imagine this system in terms of driving a car. The creatine phosphate system

is the first system to be used in the body, just like first gear is the first gear to be used in a car. If you were to drive a long distance in first gear, the amount of fuel used would be enormous and therefore not very efficient. This is the same in the body: if you used only creatine phosphate as an energy source, it would run out very quickly. The body needs to move into another system to provide energy, just like the car needs to move into second gear. However, it must be noted that all energy systems are active at the same time.

The anaerobic or lactic acid system

Glucose (without oxygen)

Glucose is a sugar found in carbohydrate foods such as potatoes, vegetables, rice, bread and fruit. When carbohydrates are digested they release glucose, which is then stored in the body as *glycogen*. Glucose in the blood or glycogen from stores in the body are then used to supply phosphates. The process of breaking down glucose to provide energy is called *anaerobic glycolysis*.

If the exercise intensity is high, this energy supply system can be maintained continuously only for two to three minutes, as it produces a substance called *lactic acid* as a waste product (see Fig. 6.4). Lactic acid can stop muscle contraction if too much is produced, and the greater the intensity of exercise, the more lactic acid is produced.

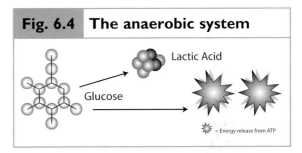

| Fig. 6.4 | **The anaerobic system** |

As this is the next system that the body uses to supply energy after the ATP–CP system, it is equivalent to using second gear in a car. If you were going on a long journey in a car, you would again use a lot of fuel if you stayed in this gear for the entire journey. It is the same in the body: only two ATP molecules are produced from each glucose molecule, so the body needs to move on to the next, more efficient system or gear.

The aerobic system

Glucose (with oxygen)

After a few minutes of exercise, oxygen is transported to the muscles to be used with glucose to provide energy in a system called *aerobic glycolysis*. As long as the intensity is not too high, and oxygen is present, there will be no build-up of lactic acid. Carbon dioxide and water are given off as waste products (see Fig. 6.5).

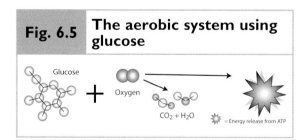

Fig. 6.5	**The aerobic system using glucose**

When oxygen is used in re-synthesis it is more efficient, as 38 molecules of ATP are produced per molecule of oxygen. However, one of the problems with this system is that there is only sufficient glycogen stored in the body for medium intensity exercise of about two hours duration, if the storage is full prior to the exercise: if glycogen stores have been used up in previous exercise and haven't yet been replaced, the possible duration of exercise using this system will be less. This is similar to going on a long journey in a car and having a less than full fuel tank – either you can't travel as far, or you need to re-fuel. Carbohydrate drinks can be taken during exercise to supply glucose to the muscles; this also spares the stores in the body. It is also important to eat a carbohydrate snack as soon as possible after exercise to replace glucose that has been used during the exercise. However, rather than rely on this system for energy, the body has another system that is even more efficient and uses fat, among other things, as a fuel.

Fat (with oxygen)

After several minutes of exercise (this time varies with fitness levels) intramuscular fat or fat that is transported to the muscle can be used in the energy process. In order for this to happen, small amounts of glucose and oxygen must be available. The place in the muscle where energy is released by breaking down fat, carbohydrate and oxygen is called the *mitochondria* (see also pages 38 and 94). There is no build-up of lactic acid, but carbon dioxide, water and heat are given off as by-products (see Fig. 6.6). This system is used when the exercise is of low-to-moderate intensity, such as walking or comfortable jogging. As this system uses a small amount of glucose, the exercise can be maintained only as long as glucose is available, usually about two hours (less if the exercise was started on low stores of glucose), unless carbohydrates are taken in during the exercise. **Note:** There are other ways to metabolise fat which are beyond the scope of this book.

Fig. 6.6	**The aerobic system using fat**

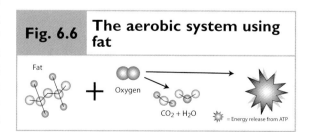

Depending on the type of fat used in this system (there are several types of fat available from food), more than 200 ATP molecules can be produced from each molecule of fat, glucose and oxygen. This makes this system very efficient in producing energy for muscle contraction. However, if stores of glucose do run out, it can be difficult for the body to break down fat. This is another reason why carbohydrate foods are important when exercising.

A person who exercises on a regular basis will move through the systems, like the gears in a car, to get to the system using fat more quickly than a person who is not used to exercise. This is simply because the body responds to the exercise regularity by becoming more efficient.

Interaction of energy systems

The body actually uses all of the above systems at the same time; however, the intensity of the exercise dictates which energy system will be used to supply the majority of the energy (see Fig. 6.7).

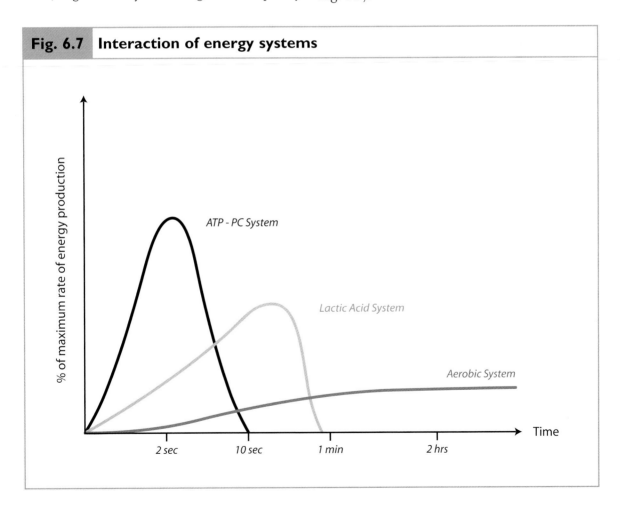

Fig. 6.7 **Interaction of energy systems**

For example, at the start of exercise (warm-up) the demand for oxygen cannot be met quickly by the aerobic system, so the anaerobic system must contribute more to energy production. However, as the warm-up continues the capillaries in the lungs and muscles dilate, increasing the flow of oxygen so that the contribution from the aerobic systems increases. After a period of time, which in some cases can be up to 30 minutes or more (at low to medium intensity), most of the energy is provided by the fat system, with the other systems providing a small amount. If, during low- to medium-intensity exercise, the individual decides to increase to a high intensity, the sudden requirement for extra energy usually comes from extra glucose in the body.

However, the problem here is that large amounts of glucose will be needed to provide the large amount of energy required to sustain the high-intensity exercise. This means that large amounts of the by-product lactic acid will be produced, which will eventually stop the muscle from contracting. High-intensity exercise producing large amounts of lactic acid is normally only sustainable for about two minutes, and much less in unfit people.

Table 6.1 shows the main energy systems used in typical sporting activities.

Table 6.1	Major energy systems used in typical activities	
Major energy system	Performance time	Typical activities
ATP–CP	<10 seconds	Shot putt 100 m sprints
Anaerobic glycolysis	20–90 seconds	200–400 m sprints Speed skating 100 m swim
Aerobic glycolysis	90 seconds to several minutes	Gymnastics 800 m run Boxing round
Fat	More than several minutes	Jogging

EXAMPLE QUESTIONS

6.1 When a phosphate molecule is split from ATP what does it leave?
a) Creatine
b) CP
c) AMP
d) ADP

6.2 What is the main process that occurs within mitochondria?
a) production of ATP without the presence of oxygen
b) production of ATP in the presence of oxygen
c) converting glucose to glycogen in the presence of oxygen
d) converting glucose to glycogen without the presence of oxygen

6.3 Anaerobic glycolysis is...
a) breaking down glucose in the presence of oxygen
b) breaking down glucose without the presence of oxygen
c) converting glucose to glycogen in the presence of oxygen
d) converting glucose to glycogen without the presence of oxygen

6.4 Aerobic glycolysis is...
a) breaking down glucose in the presence of oxygen
b) breaking down glucose without the presence of oxygen
c) converting glucose to glycogen in the presence of oxygen
d) converting glucose to glycogen without the presence of oxygen

6.5 Which of the following is given off as a by-product of aerobic glycolysis?
a) ATP
b) hydrogen
c) lactic acid
d) carbon dioxide and water

EXAMPLE QUESTIONS cont.

6.6 Which of the following is given off as a by-product of anaerobic glycolysis?
a) ATP
b) hydrogen
c) lactic acid
d) carbon dioxide and water

6.7 Which of the following is produced as a result of incomplete breakdown of fat due to lack of available carbohydrate?
a) lactic acid
b) hydrogen
c) ketones
d) carbon dioxide and water

6.8 Which energy system contributes the most (in percentage terms) at the start of exercise?
a) anaerobic glycolysis
b) aerobic glycolysis
c) ATP–PC system
d) fat

6.9 Which energy system contributes the least (in percentage terms) at the start of exercise?
a) anaerobic glycolysis
b) aerobic glycolysis
c) ATP–PC system
d) aerobic (fat)

6.10 Which energy system contributes the most (in percentage terms) in short sprint events such as the 100 metres?
a) anaerobic glycolysis
b) aerobic glycolysis
c) ATP–PC system
d) aerobic (fat)

EXAMPLE QUESTIONS cont.

6.11 Which energy system contributes the most (in percentage terms) in events such as the 800 metres?
 a) they are all the same
 b) aerobic glycolysis
 c) ATP–PC system
 d) lactic acid system

6.12 Which energy system contributes the most (in percentage terms) in events such as a long distance run?
 a) they are all the same
 b) aerobic (fat)
 c) ATP–PC system
 d) lactic acid system

Further reading

Abrahams, P., Craven, J. and Lumley, J. (2011) *Illustrated Clinical Anatomy* (2nd ed.), Hodder Arnold

Baechle, R.T. (2008) *Essentials of Strength Training and Conditioning* (3rd ed.), Human Kinetics

Gastin, P.B. (2001) 'Energy system interaction and relative contribution during maximal exercise', *Sports Medicine*, 31: 725–741

Hargreaves, M., and Spriet, L. (2006) *Exercise Metabolism*, Human Kinetics

McArdle, W.D., Katch, F.I. and Katch, V.L. (2007) *Exercise Physiology* (6th ed.), Lippincott, Williams & Wilkins

Maud, P. and Foster, C. (2006) *Physiological Assessment of Human Fitness* (2nd ed.), Human Kinetics

Mougios, V. (2006) *Exercise Biochemistry*, Human Kinetics

Porter, S. (2002) *The Anatomy Workbook*, Butterworth Heinemann

Ross, J.S. and Wilson, J.W. (2006) *Anatomy and Physiology in Health and Illness* (10th ed.), Churchill Livingstone

Sewell, D., Watkins, P. and Griffin, M. (2005) *Sport and Exercise Science: An Introduction*, Hodder Arnold

Tortora, G.J. and Grabowski, S.R. (2005) *Principles of Anatomy and Physiology* (11th ed.), Wiley

NOTES

THE HEART AND THE CIRCULATORY SYSTEM

7

OBJECTIVES

After completing this chapter, you will be able to:

1 Describe the structure of the heart in relation to the layers of muscle and surrounding sheath.

2 Name and describe the sections within the heart.

3 Explain the process of heart contraction (cardiac cycle).

4 Describe the flow of blood into and away from the heart and describe the features of the associated vessels.

5 Describe the composition of blood.

6 Explain the mechanisms of venous return.

7 Explain the terms *hypertension* and *hypotension* in relation to blood pressure and how exercise affects blood pressure.

8 The short- and long-term effects of exercise on the heart and circulation system.

9 The key cardiovascular differences in special population groups.

Level 2: Instructing Exercise and Fitness Knowledge

Basic Anatomy and Physiology
- The location and function of the heart; the function of arteries, veins and capillaries.
- The short- and long-term effects of exercise on the heart and circulation system.

Level 3: Instructing Physical Activity and Exercise Knowledge

Anatomy: Cardiovascular system
- Anatomy of the heart:
  - The four chambers
  - Valves and control of blood flow
  - The cardiac cycle
  - Conduction systems (autonomic and intrinsic)
  - Cardiac output (regulation of stroke volume and heart rate)
  - Cardiac circulation

- Structure, function and characteristics of arteries, arterioles, veins and capillaries
- Coronary circulation
- Systemic circulation
- Pathway of oxygen from inhaled air to muscle
- Pathway of carbon dioxide from muscle to exhaled air

Introduction

This chapter deals with the anatomical system of the body in relation to the cardiac and circulatory systems (known as the cardiovascular system) from the perspective of structure, function and the effects of exercise. Within the National Occupational Standards framework, Level 2 and 3 instructors should be able to describe the common structures of both systems and describe their functions, as well as describe how exercise can impact on the systems.

Later chapters in the book provide physiological and biomechanical principles that, together with the knowledge of the cardiovascular system covered in this chapter, will provide you with the understanding and ability to design appropriate exercise programmes for apparently healthy individuals and to understand the effects of various types of exercise on the human body.

The cardiopulmonary system

The system that supplies oxygen and nutrients to the muscles and takes away waste products such as carbon dioxide is called the cardiopulmonary system, and is made up of the lungs, heart and associated vessels (see Fig. 7.1). The lungs provide the system that delivers oxygen to and extracts carbon dioxide from the blood.

The heart

The heart is a cone-shaped organ about the size of a clenched fist and lies on the diaphragm, just left of the midline of the body. It provides a pumping service that maintains a constant circulation or blood flow to carry oxygen and carbon dioxide around the body. The wall of the heart is made up of three layers. The *myocardium* (*myo* meaning muscle), which is the middle layer, is the predominant layer and is essentially the heart muscle. The myocardium is covered on the inside by a layer of tissue known as the *endocardium* (*endo* meaning within) and on the outside by a layer of tissue known as the *epicardium* (*epi* meaning without). The entire heart is then surrounded by a fibrous tissue called the *pericardium* (*peri* meaning around), which is filled with fluid in order to protect and anchor the heart.

NEED TO KNOW

The heart beats about 100,000 times a day, or 35 million times a year, and pumps blood around an estimated 100,000 km of blood vessels.

The heart can be divided into left and right sides by a muscular wall known as the *septum*, which literally translates as 'dividing wall'. Each side contains an upper and a lower chamber.

Fig. 7.1   The cardiopulmonary system

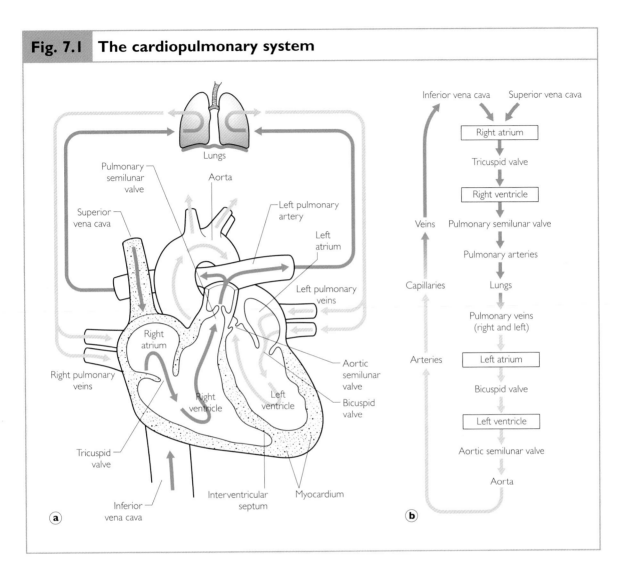

Each upper chamber is called an *atrium* (*atria* meaning entry hall) and each lower chamber is called a *ventricle* (*ventricle* meaning little belly). The left ventricle is larger and has thicker walls than the right ventricle, as it pumps blood into the arteries and has to force against the pressure of the blood exerted as the arteries become progressively smaller.

Blood flow through the heart is a one-way system controlled by a number of one-way valves. The four main valves in the heart are as follows:

Atrioventricular valves

The atrioventricular valves control the flow of blood between the atrium and ventricles. The right atrioventricular valve is called the *tricuspid valve* and the left is called the *bicuspid* or *mitral valve*.

Semi-lunar valves

As the name suggests, semi-lunar valves are in the shape of a half moon (*semi* meaning half and *lunar* meaning moon-shaped). These valves are located at the exits to arteries from the respective ventricles. The right ventricle valve, leading to the opening of the pulmonary artery, is called the *pulmonary valve* and the left ventricle valve, leading to the opening of the aorta, is called the *aortic valve*.

NEED TO KNOW

Aorte means to suspend, as it was once thought that the job of the main artery, the aorta, was to lift up the heart.

The cardiac cycle

All chambers of the heart contract and relax in a specific sequence in order to pump blood out or to fill up with blood. *Cardiac cycle* refers to this sequence of contraction and relaxation – in other words, the time taken from the start of one

---

NEED TO KNOW

Each heartbeat is stimulated by an electrical impulse that originates in a small strip of heart tissue known as the sinoatrial (S-A) node, or pacemaker.

One of the most important advances in cardiology is the electrical pacemaker. This originates the electrical impulses when the patient's is defective.

---

beat to the start of another beat. The cardiac cycle can be measured by a qualified person using an ECG machine, which produces a trace known as the PQRST wave. This is essentially the trace of electrical activity across the heart during the cardiac cycle. The electrical activity in the heart is activated subconsciously by the sinoatrial node, which is a group of specialised cells in the right atrium responsible for the ordered contraction and relaxation of the heart. The sinoatrial node is also known as the natural pacemaker.

The sequence of electrical activity across the heart during a cardiac cycle is quite quick as the heart beats on average about 72 times per minute. The number of times the heart beats every minute is called the heart rate and is measured in beats per minute (bpm). The sequence of events for the cardiac cycle is as follows:

1. The 'P' section represents the contraction of the atria (atrial systole), which pumps blood into the ventricles. At this point, the ventricles are relaxed (ventricular diastole). Electrical activity is not very high as the atria do not contract strongly; this is because they are assisted by gravity and the blood is not under a large amount of pressure.

2. The 'QRS' section represents the forceful contraction of the ventricles (ventricular systole) to pump blood through the aortic and pulmonary valves into the respective vessels. This occurs about 0.1 seconds after the contraction of the atria. At this point, the valves between the atria and ventricles are closed to prevent backflow. The amount of blood pumped out of the ventricles each beat is called the *stroke volume* and the volume of blood left in the ventricles after they have contracted is called the *end systolic volume*.

3. The 'T' section is when the ventricles are relaxed and the atria are filling up prior to

their activation. The electrical activity here is returning to a resting state.

The whole cycle lasts about 0.8 seconds.

Cardiac output

The amount of blood pumped out of the heart every minute is known as the cardiac output. This can be written as follows:

Cardiac output = heart rate × stroke volume

As heart rate is measured in beats per minute (bpm) and stroke volume is measured in millilitres (mls), cardiac output is measured in millilitres per minute (mls.min^{-1}). Exercise can make the heart grow stronger, which could result in an increase in stroke volume as the heart can pump out more blood. As sub maximal heart rate normally reduces as a long-term effect of exercise, this would mean that even though stroke volume increases, cardiac output stays relatively the same due to the reduction in heart rate.

TASK

Give a brief description of the heart and the cardiac cycle, describing any terms that you use.

Blood

Blood flow

Two *pulmonary veins* (one from each lung) carry blood that is rich in oxygen (oxygenated blood) to the left atrium in the heart. This is known as the *pulmonary circulation system*. The blood then passes through the left atrioventricular valve into the left ventricle, from where it is forcefully pumped through the aortic valve into the first (main) artery, the *aorta*.

Oxygenated blood is then pumped around a network of arteries leading to places that require it, such as muscles and organs. This is known as the *systemic circulation system*. The oxygen is passed into the muscles or organs through the smallest vessels, known as capillaries, and at the same time carbon dioxide passes from the muscles or organs into the capillaries. This exchange of gases is known as *diffusion*.

The deoxygenated blood then makes the return journey to the heart, carrying waste products such as carbon dioxide. The blood moves through a network of veins into the two main veins, called the *superior* and *inferior vena cavae*. These two veins empty the blood into the right atrium. The blood then passes through the right atrioventricular valve into the right ventricle. This process is called *venous return*.

The right ventricle then pumps the deoxygenated blood through the pulmonary valve and into the pulmonary artery. This leads back to the lungs, where carbon dioxide passes out of the capillaries into the lungs and oxygen is diffused back into the capillaries to be taken back to the left atrium via the pulmonary vein. The journey the blood makes from the right ventricle via the lungs to the left atrium is known as *pulmonary circulation*. The process then starts again. For more information on the function of the lungs, see Chapter 8.

The composition of blood

Blood is made up of straw-coloured transparent fluid called *plasma* and different types of cells that are suspended in the plasma. Typically, blood contains about 55 per cent plasma and 45 per cent cells. The two types of cells within blood are known as red and white blood cells.

Red blood cells

Otherwise known as *erythrocytes*, red blood cells are made in the bone marrow and last for about 120 days, circulating within the body. Red blood cells contain a protein known as *haemoglobin*, which is responsible for combining with oxygen or carbon dioxide to transport it through the bloodstream. When haemoglobin combines with oxygen, it is known as *oxyhaemoglobin*; when carbon dioxide is transported in the blood, it is known as *carbaminohaemoglobin*.

White blood cells

Otherwise known as *leukocytes*, white blood cells are the largest of the blood cells and account for about 1 per cent of the total blood volume. The main function of white blood cells is to protect the body against any foreign bodies and to remove any waste material, called *cell debris*. There are many different types of leukocytes, which have specific roles within the body.

Platelets

These are very small discs made in the red bone marrow that have a lifespan of between 8 and 11 days. Platelets help to prevent blood loss when a blood vessel is damaged. First, they are involved in vasoconstriction of the vessel at the damaged site and then in plugging the break. They are then involved in blood clotting at the site of the damage. When all of this occurs, the damage to the vessel can be repaired and breakdown of the clot can begin.

The circulation system

Within the body is a network of vessels known as arteries, veins and capillaries that carry the blood and its contents to all areas. These vessels each have different functions and structures.

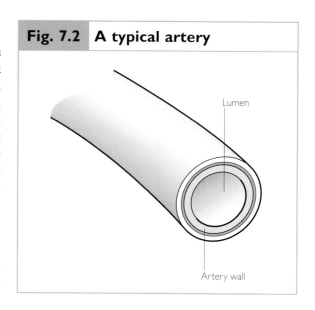

Fig. 7.2 | **A typical artery**

Lumen

Artery wall

Arteries

Arteries carry oxygenated blood that is under pressure away from the heart. Arteries are round with thick, elastic, muscular walls to withstand the pressure. Because of the muscular walls, arteries can get narrower (*vasoconstriction*) or open up (*vasodilation*). The space inside the artery is known as the lumen. In cases of heart disease, the lumen can become blocked by fatty deposits (*atherosclerosis*), which can then restrict blood flow and increase blood pressure. See Fig. 7.2.

Arteries close to the heart are thicker than those further away due to the increased pressure they have to withstand. As the arteries branch out away from the heart, they become smaller and are known as *arterioles*. As they branch out even further, they become minute vessels called *capillaries* (see pages 109–10).

Veins

Veins carry the blood back to the heart once it has delivered oxygen to the sites that require it. In other words, veins carry deoxygenated blood. The veins are not as round as arteries

Fig. 7.3 A typical vein

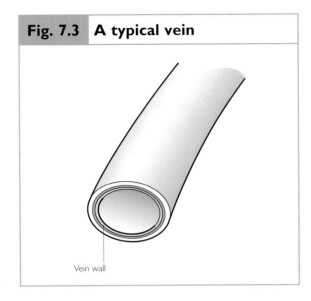

Vein wall

Gravity

Any blood that is above the level of the heart is assisted by gravity to help it return to the heart.

Muscle contraction

Skeletal muscle contraction and smooth muscle peristaltic action help to pump blood back to the heart.

Breathing

Breathing increases pressure in the abdominal cavity, which assists blood flow back to the heart.

Capillaries

Capillaries are the smallest vessels of both arteries and veins. They are only one cell thick and porous so that carbon dioxide, oxygen and other substances can pass through in a process called *gaseous exchange*. However, red blood cells cannot pass through the capillary walls. See Fig. 7.4.

and have thinner walls, as there is less pressure on them. See Fig. 7.3.

Oxygenated blood flows through arteries then passes into arterioles then capillaries. The de-oxygenated blood (having given up its oxygen) then flows into vessels called venules, which in turn then flow into larger vessels called veins. As the blood that veins carry is not under as much pressure as that carried by the arteries, the veins need a system (known as venous return) to prevent a possible backflow of blood which could lead to an effect called *blood pooling* which is essentially an inefficient return of de-oxygenated blood back to the heart. This would certainly reduce the capacity for exercise and might also cause dizziness and fatigue. Veins therefore have a series of one-way valves that prevent the blood from flowing backwards against the normal direction of blood flow. These one-way valves can get damaged due to high blood pressure or disease which can have the effect of reducing venous return. Other mechanisms that contribute to venous return are gravity, muscle contraction and breathing.

Fig. 7.4 A typical capillary

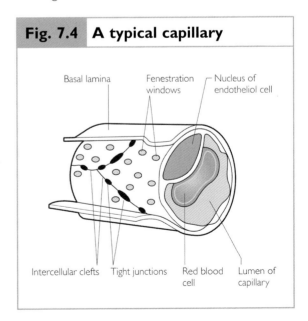

Basal lamina

Fenestration windows

Nucleus of endotheliol cell

Intercellular clefts   Tight junctions   Red blood cell   Lumen of capillary

Thousands of capillaries wrap around muscles so that oxygen can be delivered and carbon dioxide extracted. At the start of a network, before they branch out, capillaries have muscular sphincters (round muscles) that can open or close to either allow or prevent blood flow to the network (sometimes called *blood shunting*). These are used to ensure the areas of the body that need it the most receive oxygen at the expense of other areas. For example, when there is an increased demand for oxygen by muscles during exercise, capillary sphincters will open at the muscles doing the exercise and close in places such as the digestive system where oxygen is not required.

TASK

Describe the composition of blood, the vessels that carry the blood and the method by which oxygen circulates around the body.

Blood pressure and exercise

Pressure is needed to pump the blood around the body otherwise it would simply gravitate to the lowest parts of the body. The pressure is greatest at the aorta, as the left ventricle forcefully pumps the blood through it. By the time the blood reaches the capillaries, it is still under pressure, but not as much as in the aorta.

There are two phases of blood pressure: *systolic* and *diastolic*. Systolic pressure is the pressure on the artery walls when the ventricles contracts and diastolic pressure is the pressure on the artery walls when the ventricles fill between beats.

The two phases of pressure can be measured to evaluate if an individual is within safe limits. The American College of Sports Medicine recommends that an average of two or more readings be taken when testing blood pressure. Table 7.1 shows the ranges for normal and high blood pressure.

If blood pressure goes above or below the normal range, it is deemed to be high or low respectively. High blood pressure is known as *hypertension* and low blood pressure is known as *hypotension*.

Hypertension

High blood pressure can be caused by various factors, but regardless of the cause, the rate of the heart and force at which it contracts are increased to maintain the amount of blood

Table 7.1	Ranges for normal and high blood pressure	
	Systolic	Diastolic
Normal	< 120 and	< 80
Pre-hypertension	120–139 or	80–89
Hypertension (stage 1)	140–159 or	90–99
Hypertension (stage 2)	≥ 160–179 or	≥100–109

Adapted from the ACSM GETP (2006)

required by the body. Long-term hypertension can result in heart attack or stroke.

During a bout of exercise, systolic blood pressure tends to rise whereas diastolic blood pressure stays about the same (and can even decrease slightly). Regular low-intensity aerobic exercise has been shown to reduce both systolic and diastolic blood pressure. Exercise can also prevent the tendency for blood pressure to rise in the long term. This preventative measure is important, as there is less risk of heart disease in individuals who have never been hypertensive.

Hypotension

Hypotension refers to blood pressure below the normal range. Although the effects are not the same as in hypertension, individuals who have lower than normal blood pressure should be advised to move slowly when coming from a floor position to a standing position. This is because the low blood pressure can cause a reduction in blood flow to the brain due to gravity, which can cause fainting.

NEED TO KNOW

People with hypertension should avoid isometric or heavy resistance exercises as they can elevate blood pressure. Also, trying to perform and exercise whilst attempting a forceful exhalation against a closed airway (glotis) is not recommended as this could cause an increase in blood pressure. This is known as the *Valsalva manoeuvre*.

The effects of exercise on the heart

Short-term effects

Exercise leads to an increase in the rate of *cardiac output* (CO). The stroke volume is also increased, as the heart is pumping faster to supply oxygenated blood to the working muscles.

Long-term effects

The long-term effects of exercise on the heart include the following:

1. An increase in the size and strength of the cardiac muscle.
2. An increase in venous return, which reduces blood pooling.
3. Working (systolic) and resting (diastolic) blood pressure lowers, enabling the heart to work more efficiently.
4. The resting and sub-maximal heart rate decreases.
5. Stroke volume increases.

The effects of exercise on the circulation system

Short-term effects

The short-term effects of exercise on the circulation system include the following:

1. Blood is diverted from non-essential areas (for example the digestive system) to the muscles that are being used.
2. Some blood vessels narrow (vasoconstrict) and some widen (vasodilate).

Long-term effects

The long-term effects of exercise on the circulation system include the following:

1. An improvement in general circulation.
2. Vasoconstriction and vasodilation become more efficient.
3. The number of capillaries and mitochondria increases.
4. Greater quantities of red blood cells are produced in order to meet the requirements for an increase in the oxygen-carrying capacity of the blood.
5. There are increased levels of haemoglobin in the blood to increase the blood's capacity to bind and transport oxygen to the working muscles.

Key cardiovascular differences between special population groups

Instructors should be aware that there are cardiovascular differences between an apparently healthy population and special population groups (children/young people, older adults and ante/postnatal). Table 7.2 outlines the main differences and the implications for exercise.

Table 7.2	Cardiovascular differences between special population groups	
Special population group	Main cardiovascular differences	Exercise implication
Children/young people	Walking/running economy is less Cardiac output and stroke volume lower Thermoregulation not as efficient Higher maximum heart rate	Perform extended warm-up / cool downs and limit duration of higher intensity activities. Avoid extremes of temperature and keep well hydrated especially in winter. Always supervise exercises.
Older adults	Cardiac output, stroke volume, VO_2max and heart rate decrease. Blood pressure increases.	Any progression should be slow and to individual capacity. Get regular feedback during and after exercise. Introduce post-exercise relaxation. Avoid fatigue. Use cycling and swimming for those with reduced weight-bearing capacity.
Ante/postnatal	Increase in resting heart rate. Decrease in venous return. Cardiac output increases. Left ventricle and blood vessels enlarge. Blood flow to the skin increases.	Avoid motionless or exercise in the supine position. Be aware of heating up quickly. Limit higher intensity to short periods. No high impact and no exhaustion. Low intensity only (after medical approval) if there is no history of exercise. Stop if any pain or discomfort.

EXAMPLE QUESTIONS

7.1 The heart muscle is divided into left and right sides by what?
a) endocardium
b) epicardium
c) mitrum
d) septum

7.2 The heart muscle is entirely covered by a layer of fibrous tissue known as what?
a) pericardium
b) epicardium
c) endocardium
d) myocardium

7.3 The term 'entry hall' relates to which structure in the heart?
a) sino-atrial node
b) ventricle
c) atrium
d) aorta

7.4 The mitral valve is otherwise known as the what?
a) aortic
b) tri-cuspid
c) bi-cuspid
d) semilunar

7.5 The sino-atrial node can be found in which chamber of the heart?
a) right atrium
b) left atrium
c) right ventricle
d) left ventricle

EXAMPLE QUESTIONS cont.

7.6 The aortic valve can be found leading from which chamber of the heart?

a) right atrium

b) left atrium

c) right ventricle

d) left ventricle

7.7 The amount of blood pumped out of the ventricles each beat is known as what?

a) end diastolic volume

b) cardiac output

c) stroke volume

d) residual volume

7.8 The amount of blood pumped out of the ventricles each beat, multiplied by the heart rate in beats per minute is known as what?

a) end diastolic volume

b) cardiac output

c) stroke volume

d) residual volume

7.9 The amount of blood left in the ventricles after each beat is known as what?

a) end diastolic volume

b) cardiac output

c) stroke volume

d) residual volume

7.10 Which of the following protect the body against foreign bodies?

a) white blood cells

b) red blood cells

c) plasma

d) platelets

EXAMPLE QUESTIONS cont.

7.11 Which of the following help in blood clotting?

a) red blood cells

b) platelets

c) plasma

d) white blood cells

7.12 Blood pressure is greatest in which vessel?

a) pulmonary artery

b) pulmonary vein

c) aorta

d) vena cava

Further reading

Abrahams, P., Craven, J. and Lumley, J. (2011) *Illustrated Clinical Anatomy* (2nd ed.), Hodder Arnold

American College of Obstetricians and Gynecologists (2002) 'ACOG Committee Opinion No.267: Exercise during pregnancy and the postpartum period', *Obstetrics and Gynecology*, 99: 171–173

American College of Sports Medicine (2006) *Guidelines to Exercise Testing and Prescription* (7th ed.), Lippincott, Williams & Wilkins

American Congress of Obstetricians and Gynecologists (2003) *Exercise During Pregnancy*, ACOG

Baechle, R.T. (2008) *Essentials of Strength Training and Conditioning* (3rd ed.), Human Kinetics

Fitzgerald, M.D., Tanaka, H., Tran, Z.V. and Seals, D.R. (1997) 'Age-related declines in maximal aerobic capacity in regularly exercising vs. sedentary women: a meta-analysis', *Journal of Applied Physiology*, 83: 160–165

Kubukeli, Z.N., Noakes, T.D. and Dennis, S.C. (2002) 'Training techniques to improve endurance exercise performances', *Sports Medicine* 32: 489–509

Marieb, E.N. (2009) *Human Anatomy and Physiology* (8th ed.), Benjamin Cummings Publishing Company Inc.

McArdle, W.D., Katch, F.I. and Katch, V.L. (2007) *Exercise Physiology* (6th ed.), Lippincott, Williams & Wilkins

Paisley, T.S., Joy, E.A., & Price, R.J. (2003) 'Exercise during pregnancy: a practical approach', *Current Sports Medicine Reports*, 2: 325–330

Pendergast, D.R., Fisher, N.M. and Calkins, E. (1993) 'Cardiovascular, neuromuscular and metabolic alterations with age leading to frailty', *Journal of Gerontology*, 48: 61–67

Porter, S. (2002) *The Anatomy Workbook*, Butterworth Heinemann

Ross, J.S. and Wilson, J.W. (2006) *Anatomy and Physiology in Health and Illness* (10th ed.), Churchill Livingstone

Sewell, D., Watkins, P. and Griffin, M. (2005) *Sport and Exercise Science: An introduction*, Hodder Arnold

Tortora, G.J. and Grabowski, S.R. (2005) *Principles of Anatomy and Physiology* (11th ed.), Wiley

Twisk, J. (2001) 'Physical activity guidelines for children and adolescents: a critical review', *Sports Medicine*, 31: 617–627

Wilmore, J.H. and Costhill, D.L. (2011) *Physiology of Sport and Exercise* (5th ed.), Human Kinetics

NOTES

THE RESPIRATORY SYSTEM

OBJECTIVES

After completing this chapter, you will be able to:

1 Describe the structure of the lungs in relation to their function.

2 Explain the passage of air into and out of the lungs.

3 Explain the process of exchange of gases.

4 List the percentages of gases in inspired and expired air.

5 Explain the mechanism of breathing.

6 The short and long term effects of exercise on the respiratory system.

7 The key respiratory differences in special population groups.

Level 2: Instructing Exercise and Fitness Knowledge

Basic Anatomy and Physiology

■ The location and function of the lungs and capillaries.

■ The short- and long-term effects of exercise on the respiratory system.

Level 3: Instructing Physical Activity and Exercise Knowledge

Anatomy: The Respiratory System

■ Anatomy of the lungs:

  • Structure of the lungs and airways
  • Inspiration and expiration (including the role of the diaphragm and intercostal muscles)
  • Breathing regulation (respiratory centre – hypothalamus)
  • Effect of smoking on the lungs

■ Pathway of oxygen from inhaled air to muscle

■ Pathway of carbon dioxide from muscle to exhaled air

Introduction

This chapter deals with the anatomical system of the body in relation to the respiratory system from the perspective of structure, function and the effects of exercise. Within the National Occupational Standards framework, Level 2 and 3 instructors should be able to describe the common structures of the respiratory system and describe the function of the system, as well as describe how exercise can impact on the system.

Later chapters in the book provide physiological and biomechanical principles that, together with the knowledge of the cardiovascular system covered in the previous chapter and the respiratory system covered in this chapter, provide you with the understanding and ability to design appropriate exercise programmes for apparently healthy individuals and to understand the effects of various types of exercise on the human body.

The respiratory system

The *respiratory system* is the collective term given to the nose, pharynx, larynx, trachea, bronchi and lungs. Essentially, it filters, warms and moistens air before conducting it to the lungs, which house specific sites where gases are exchanged between the air and the blood. See Fig. 8.1.

The lungs

The lungs are a pair of cone-shaped organs made of elastic tissue that expand to allow air from the atmosphere to enter. They are roughly level with the heart in the thoracic cavity and are surrounded by a double membrane called the *pleura*. Each lung has a superior (upper), middle and inferior (lower) lobe.

Fig. 8.1 The respiratory system

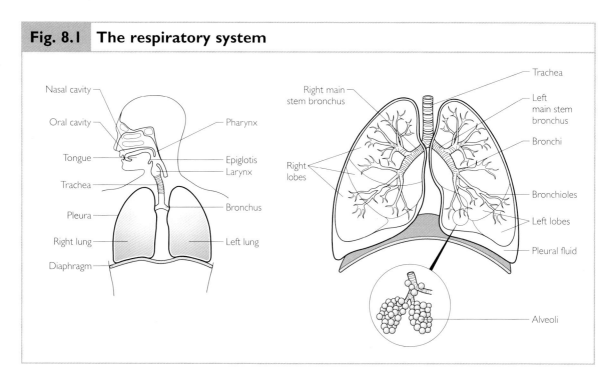

The passage of air

Air that is breathed in is known as *inspired air*, while air that is breathed out is called *expired air*. Air is made up of various gases, and the composition of gases in inspired air is different from that of expired air (see Table 8.1). About 5 per cent of the oxygen in inspired air is used up, so expired air contains less oxygen. About 4 per cent carbon dioxide is produced during breathing, so expired air has more carbon dioxide than inspired air.

The *passage of air* describes how oxygen from the air reaches the muscles that require it for the production of energy. First, air is taken in through the mouth or the nose. If the air is passed through the nose, it can be warmed, moistened and filtered; this occurs to a lesser extent to air taken in through the mouth, which can induce asthmatic reactions. The air then passes through the *pharynx* (throat), which lies behind the nose and the mouth and is a passage for food and air. The pharynx is lined with a mucous membrane that provides moisture, and the wall of the pharynx is made of skeletal muscle (see pages 39–40). The pharynx also houses the tonsils, which play a part in reactions against foreign invaders such as viruses.

The air then passes down through the *larynx* (voice box), which extends to the level of the start of the thoracic vertebrae. The air is continually warmed and moistened as it travels through the larynx. The larynx wall is made up of several

pieces of cartilage connected by muscle tissue. One of the pieces of cartilage is known as the *epiglottis* (*epi* meaning over and *glottis* meaning tongue), which is essentially a trapdoor that controls the passage of air and food (it closes when swallowing to prevent food and drink going into the airways). From the larynx, the air continues into a rigid cartilaginous tube called the *trachea* (*trachea* meaning sturdy) or windpipe, which is lined with fine hairs that filter the air. The trachea runs down to the level of the fifth thoracic vertebra, where it divides into the left and right *bronchi*.

NEED TO KNOW

The thyroid cartilage is a small piece of cartilage at the front of the throat, otherwise known as the Adam's apple. Its role is to influence the tension of the vocal cords and is usually larger in males, which is why men have deeper voices than women.

Air passes into each of the bronchi, which enter the left and right lungs and split into smaller bronchi. These then split into smaller tubes called *bronchioles*, which in turn branch out and finally lead into air sacs called *alveoli*. The alveoli then fill up with air and expand to a size dependant on breathing levels and other physical factors.

Table 8.1	Composition of inspired and expired air	
	Inspired air (%)	Expired air (%)
Oxygen	21	16
Carbon dioxide	0.04	4
Nitrogen	78	78

It is here that gaseous exchange takes place, so that oxygen can enter the bloodstream to be transported to working muscles and carbon dioxide can be removed from the bloodstream in expired air. The amount of air remaining in the lungs after a maximal breath out is known as the *residual volume*.

NEED TO KNOW

Sometimes the airflow through the trachea can become blocked. Therefore, an incision is made through the wall of the trachea and a tube inserted so that the patient can breathe. This is known as a tracheotomy.

Fig. 8.2	Gaseous exchange at the alveoli

Blood in

Alveoli

CO_2 out

O_2 in

Blood out

Gaseous exchange

In order for oxygen to pass from the alveoli into the bloodstream, it must first pass through the walls of the alveoli. All alveoli are surrounded by numerous capillaries, which then lead into the network of veins and arteries. Oxygen can pass through the membrane wall of the alveoli and through the wall of the capillaries, as both structures are only one cell thick. Carbon dioxide passes the opposite way, from the capillaries into the alveoli, to be breathed out (see Fig. 8.2.).

This exchange of gases is possible due to the *pressure gradient*. In general terms, gases pass from an area of high concentration (or pressure) to an area of low concentration in order to equalise the concentration. For example, after breathing in (*inspiration*) there is a higher concentration of oxygen in the alveoli than in the capillaries surrounding them, so the oxygen diffuses from the alveoli to the capillaries. Likewise, there is a higher concentration of carbon dioxide in the capillaries than in the

alveoli, so the carbon dioxide diffuses from the capillaries into the alveoli.

Breathing control

One of the main factors involved in breathing control is the level of carbon dioxide in the blood. When the amount of carbon dioxide in the blood reaches a certain level, respiratory centres in the brain stem activate breathing muscles via the central nervous system.

Generally, the breathing rate (the number of breaths per minute) is about 12 times per minute. This increases during exercise, as the demand for more oxygen by the working muscles is recognised by the respiratory centre in the brain stem, which in turn increases the number of breaths per minute. Therefore, in this way the breathing rate is controlled subconsciously. Breathing can also be controlled consciously.

The amount of air taken into the lungs during a normal breath is called the *tidal volume*. The maximum amount of air breathed out after a maximal inspiration is called the *vital capacity* and is sometimes measured to monitor progress during an exercise programme although it is mainly used to identify possible lung disease.

The role of muscles in breathing

The main muscles involved in breathing in (inspiration) when an individual is not involved in exercise are the diaphragm and the external intercostals. The scalenes and the pectoralis minor contribute during vigorous exercise. Essentially when the inspiratory muscles contract, the diaphragm has the effect of pulling the ribcage down and expanding the thorax area which results in drawing air in as the pressure of the lungs that have stretched is less than the air pressure outside the body. This is called a pressure gradient.

Expiration (breathing out) is predominantly passive, as the result of *elastic recoil* by certain tissues: tissues such as muscles have a certain amount of elasticity, which means they will return to their pre-stretched state when the contraction stops. The muscles involved in expiration are the internal intercostals and certain abdominal muscles. During forced expiration (breathing heavily), the transversus abdominis is also used.

NEED TO KNOW

When your tummy aches after laughing forcefully it is usually due to fatigue of the transversus abdominis, which is not used to working so hard.

TASK

List and describe the structures of the respiratory system and explain how oxygen and carbon dioxide are exchanged between the air and the blood.

The effects of smoking on the respiratory system

The exact mechanisms of the effects of smoking on the respiratory system are complicated and are still being investigated in current research. However, a summary of the effects is given below.

1. Tar from cigarettes can remain in the alveoli, which can restrict the amount of air taken in.
2. Cigarette smoke can destroy the alveoli wall, which prevents the diffusion of oxygen and carbon dioxide.
3. Smoking is one of the leading causes of chronic bronchitis, which is the inflammation of the airways leading to a restriction in the passage of air.
4. Smoking is one of the most common causes of lung cancer. Most people with lung cancer die within the first year of diagnosis.
5. Pneumonia, which relates to inflammation of the alveoli, can be caused by smoking.
6. Nicotine from cigarettes narrows the smaller airways, which can decrease the airflow.
7 Haemoglobin (the oxygen carrier in the blood) prefers to carry carbon monoxide from smoke rather than oxygen, which reduces its oxygen-carrying capacity.
8. Smoking can cause increased mucus secretion and destroy the lining of the airways.

The effects of exercise on the respiratory system

Short-term effects

The short-term effects of exercise on the respiratory system include the following:

1. The rate of exchange of gases within the lungs increases, as does the volume of gases exchanged.
2. Levels of carbon dioxide in the body increase, so more has to be removed.
3. The depth of breathing increases, followed by the rate of breathing.

Long-term effects

The long-term effects of exercise on the respiratory system include the following:

1. The respiratory muscles become stronger.
2. Gaseous exchange at the alveoli takes place more easily.
3. The breathing effort required decreases.
4. The number of capillaries increases.
5. Tidal volume and vital capacity can increase.

Key respiratory differences between special population groups

Instructors should be aware that there are respiratory differences between an 'apparently healthy' population and special population groups (children/young people, older adults and ante/postnatal). Table 8.2 outlines the main differences and the implications for exercise.

Table 8.2	Respiratory differences between special population groups	
Special population group	**Main cardiovascular differences**	**Exercise implication**
Children/young people	Higher breathing rate (ventilation).	Children have to breathe faster for any given intensity so reduce the duration of high intensity exercise.
Older adults	Lung capacity and forced expiratory volume decrease due to muscle weakness and loss of alveoli elasticity. Maximal ventilation decreases.	Reduce intensity of exercise due to shortness of breath.
Ante/postnatal	Higher breathing rate (ventilation) as a result of increased sensitivity to carbon dioxide. Decreased residual volume. Increased oxygen consumption. Hyperventilation can occur.	Reduce intensity of exercise due to shortness of breath (even at low intensity). Be aware that hyperventilation can occur.

EXAMPLE QUESTIONS

8.1 What structures lead directly into the alveoli?

a) bronchioles

b) pleura

c) capillaries

d) bronchi

8.2 The double membrane surrounding the lungs is known as what?

a) alveoli

b) pleura

c) bronchioles

d) capillaries

8.3 The passage of oxygen and carbon dioxide in and out of the alveoli is known as what?

a) gaseous exchange

b) pressure gradient

c) elastic recoil

d) passage of air

8.4 What is the percentage of oxygen in the air that is inspired?

a) 17

b) 5

c) 21

d) 78

8.5 The amount of air left in the lungs after a breath out is known as what?

a) expiratory ratio

b) tidal volume

c) residual volume

d) vital capacity

EXAMPLE QUESTIONS cont.

8.6 The maximum amount of air breathed out of the lungs after a maximum breath in is known as what?

a) expiratory ratio

b) tidal volume

c) residual volume

d) vital capacity

8.7 Which of the following gases stimulates breathing when blood levels reach a certain point?

a) oxygen

b) carbon dioxide

c) nitrogen

d) hydrogen

8.8 The amount of air taken into the lungs during a normal breath is called what?

a) expiratory ratio

b) tidal volume

c) residual volume

d) vital capacity

8.9 Smoking is thought to be one of the main causes of what?

a) chronic bronchitis

b) heart attack

c) high cholesterol

d) obesity

8.10 Inflammation of the alveoli is otherwise known as what?

a) emphysema

b) bronchitis

c) pneumonia

d) pleurisy

EXAMPLE QUESTIONS cont.

8.11 Normal expiration is brought about as a result of what effect?

a) muscle contraction

b) gaseous exchange

c) pressure gradient

d) elastic recoil

8.12 Which is the main muscle involved in forced expiration?

a) multifidus

b) rectus abdominis

c) diaphragm

d) transversus abdominis

Further reading

Abrahams, P., Craven, J. and Lumley, J. (2011) *Illustrated Clinical Anatomy* (2nd ed.), Hodder Arnold

American College of Obstetricians and Gynecologists (2002) 'ACOG Committee Opinion No.267: Exercise during pregnancy and the postpartum period', *Obstetrics and Gynecology*, 99: 171–173

American Congress of Obstetricians and Gynecologists (2003) *Exercise During Pregnancy*, ACOG

Baechle, R.T. (2008) *Essentials of Strength Training and Conditioning* (3rd ed.), Human Kinetics

Fitzgerald, M.D., Tanaka, H., Tran, Z.V. and Seals, D.R. (1997) 'Age-related declines in maximal aerobic capacity in regularly exercising vs. sedentary women: a meta-analysis', *Journal of Applied Physiology*, 83: 160–165

Marieb, E.N. (2009) *Human Anatomy and Physiology* (8th ed.), Benjamin Cummings Publishing Company Inc.

McArdle, W.D., Katch, F.I. and Katch, V.L. (2007) *Exercise Physiology* (6th ed.), Lippincott, Williams & Wilkins

Paisley, T.S., Joy, E.A. and Price, R.J. (2003) 'Exercise during pregnancy: a practical approach', *Current Sports Medicine Reports*, 2: 325–330

Porter, S. (2002) *The Anatomy Workbook*, Butterworth Heinemann

Ross, J.S. and Wilson, J.W. (2006) *Anatomy and Physiology in Health and Illness* (10th ed.), Churchill Livingstone

Sewell, D., Watkins, P. and Griffin, M. (2005) *Sport and Exercise Science: An Introduction*, Hodder Arnold

Tortora, G.J. and Grabowski, S.R. (2005) *Principles of Anatomy and Physiology* (11th ed.), Wiley

Twisk, J. (2001) 'Physical activity guidelines for children and adolescents: a critical review', *Sports Medicine*, 31: 617–627

Wilmore, J.H. and Costhill, D.L. (2011) *Physiology of Sport and Exercise* (5th ed.), Human Kinetics

NOTES

CORE STABILITY

OBJECTIVES

After completing this chapter, you will be able to:

1 Define the terms 'stabiliser' and 'mobiliser' in relation to muscle roles.

2 Identify muscles known as local and global.

3 List the methods of spinal stabilisation.

4 Define 'neutral zone' and explain the teaching methods related to this.

5 Explain the principle of intra-abdominal pressure.

6 Describe the process for the contraction of the transversus abdominis.

7 List and describe common stability exercises.

8 Discuss exercise guidelines related to core stability.

Level 2: Instructing Exercise and Fitness Knowledge

Basic Anatomy and Physiology

■ The structure and range of movement of the spine.

■ The types of muscular contraction; location and action of major muscle groups; how voluntary muscles contract.

■ The effect of speed on posture, alignment and intensity.

■ The needs and potential of the participant, including reasons for and barriers to participation in the appropriate activity.

■ Exercises that are safe and appropriate for participants, including alternatives to potentially harmful exercises; safe and effective alignment of exercise positions.

■ Reasons for temporary deferral of exercise; referral; informed consent.

Level 3: Instructing Physical Activity and Exercise Knowledge

Anatomy: Functional Kinesiology

■ Postural muscles and core stability

■ Anatomy of muscular and mechanical systems associated with core stability:

  • Local and global stabilising muscles
  • Fibre type overview of local and global muscles

■ Fundamental principles of core stabilisation

  • Rationale for stabilisation to exist because of excessive forces on the spine
  • Neutral zone control from the muscular system
  • Intra-abdominal pressure and its role in stabilisation
  • Thoracolumbar fascia and its role in stabilisation
  • Abdominal bracing and its role in stabilisation
  • The glute complex and its role in stabilisation of the spine and reducing the risk of low back pain
  • The use of stabilisation equipment

■ Exercises associated with core stabilisation:

  • Methods of contraction of the transversus abdominis
  • Methods of abdominal bracing
  • Stability equipment exercises
  • Floor based exercises
  • Reasons for participant exclusion

Introduction

This chapter deals with the anatomical system of the body, in particular the structure and function of muscles associated with spinal stability. The chapter also deals with commonly prescribed exercises for short- and long-term development of the associated muscles. Within the National Occupational Standards framework, Level 2 and 3 instructors should be able to identify the muscular system associated with spinal, or core, stabilisation and describe their functions, as well as describe how exercise can impact on efficiency and development.

Other chapters in the book provide some of the physiological and biomechanical principles that, together with the specific theory covered in this chapter, will provide you with the understanding and ability to design appropriate exercise programmes for apparently healthy individuals and to understand the effects of various types of exercise on the human body.

Core stability

In simple terms, core stability is the process of holding the shoulder and pelvic girdles (that is, the centre part, or core of the body) stable in order to support the movement forces from the arms and legs which in turn will also increase the ability to balance. In order to do this, the muscles that are responsible for the stabilising role must function correctly in order that the muscles responsible for movement are able to perform their function correctly. Unfortunately, in many people the muscles responsible for stabilising and movement have become less than efficient due to a number of factors associated with poor posture. Everyday tasks such as sitting in cars, at desks and on sofas have led to the stabilising muscles becoming weaker, as the objects we sit on take on the role of stabilising and support. As a result, other muscles that are usually associated with movement tasks take on the role of stabilisation. This can lead to weakness in certain movements and can eventually cause muscle, tendon or ligament injury, especially in cases where the speed of a movement is increased. In turn, this will increase the possibility of injury due to the greater demand for stabilisation.

NEED TO KNOW

Everybody is capable of a certain degree of core stabilisation. However, in most cases specific muscles need to be re-trained to perform the role that they are physiologically best suited for.

Stabilisers and mobilisers

The everyday demands placed on the posture and control of the human body mean that the muscles responsible for core stabilisation (*stabilisers*, also known as *tonic muscles*) are designed to perform endurance tasks rather than short-term or explosive tasks. These muscles are sometimes described as 'nature's corset' and are required to carry out a stabilising role for long periods of time. Due to the demands of these endurance-type tasks, stabilisers are predominantly made up of type I slow-twitch fibres (see pages 44–5).

In a normal functional person, while the role of stabilisation is being undertaken muscles known as *mobilisers* are able to carry out their role of locomotion or movement of the body. These muscles are usually required to provide a short-term or *phasic* role, and are therefore not classed as endurance muscles. Mobiliser muscles are often found to be predominantly made up of fast-twitch fibres and are more superficial (closer to the surface) than stabiliser muscles.

It is commonplace for stabilising and mobilising muscles to be trained in the opposite role from that which they were designed for. For example, the rectus abdominis is predominantly a fast-twitch muscle close to the surface of the body and is normally active in strength or explosive tasks, such as running and jumping where the legs come towards the torso (spinal flexion). However, it is common for exercise programmes to include sit-up type exercises that are performed repetitively in an endurance-type capacity. The rectus abdominis is mainly responsible for this sit-up action, which effectively results in a predominantly fast-twitch muscle taking on the role of a slow-twitch muscle. This often weakens the stabiliser muscles, as the rectus abdominis has taken on this role. The drawback of this is that the rectus abdominis tries to perform both stabilising and mobilising roles, potentially leading to back pain or injury as optimal stabilisation of the spine is not performed. This reversal of roles is a common problem in exercise programmes for many different muscles within the body.

NEED TO KNOW

Lack of (or too much) flexibility in muscles can also affect their ability to either stabilise or mobilise.

Inner and outer units

Current research seems to suggest that both deep and superficial muscles in the trunk and pelvic region contribute in some way to spinal stabilisation (Richardson et al., 2003). What is not clear is the extent to which the general population has limited function of one or both of the systems.

Muscles in the body that are deep are sometimes referred to as *local muscles* or, in relation to core stabilisation, as the *inner unit*. The transversus abdominis, multifidus, pelvic floor, diaphragm and internal obliques are all examples of local muscles. Muscles that are superficial are commonly known as *global muscles* or the *outer unit*. The rectus abdominis, external obliques and some parts of the erector spinae are all global muscles. At the hip joint, the gluteus maximus and gluteus minimus are usually considered to be mobilisers and the gluteus medius is normally considered to be a stabiliser. There are many other muscles associated with stabilisation of the hip complex, but the main ones are mentioned above. The main muscles of the inner unit are listed below.

Transversus abdominis

This muscle forms a belt or corset around the trunk region and lies deep below the rectus abdominis muscle, which is associated with the 'six-pack'. Imagine a belt running underneath the navel, right around the body. This is the transversus abdominis muscle. See Fig. 9.1.

Multifidus

This is a series of many small muscles that attach between each vertebra of the spine (see Fig. 9.2.). These muscles act as a kind of lashing for the bones in the spine to prevent any excessive movement.

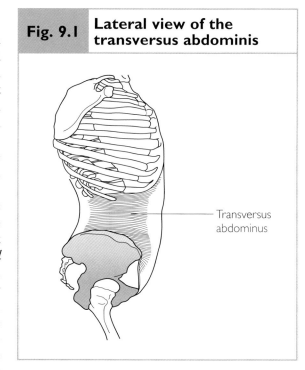

Fig. 9.1 | **Lateral view of the transversus abdominis**

Transversus abdominus

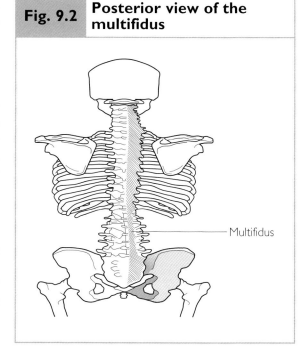

Fig. 9.2 | **Posterior view of the multifidus**

Multifidus

Internal obliques

These attach from the lower ribs and insert into the pubic bone, and lie at an angle just above and below the navel (see Fig. 9.3). They are quite deep and cannot be seen superficially.

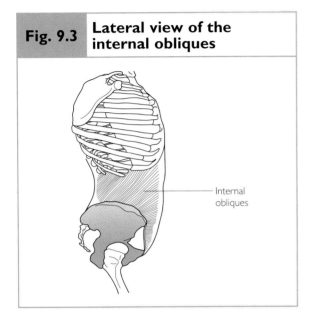

| Fig. 9.3 | **Lateral view of the internal obliques** |

Internal obliques

Pelvic floor

The pelvic floor muscles run from the coccyx (bones at the bottom of the spine), under the crotch area to the pubic bone at the front (see Fig. 9.4).

Diaphragm

This is a dome-shaped muscle that covers the region under the ribcage (see Fig. 9.5). As well as performing core stabilisation tasks, the diaphragm is responsible for helping in breathing movements.

The inner unit or local muscles are predominantly slow-twitch (tonic) and are responsible for stabilising the core of the body, in particular the spine. The outer unit or global muscles are predominantly fast-twitch (phasic) and are mainly responsible for movement, although they do contribute in a limited way to stabilisation. The main muscles of the outer unit are described below.

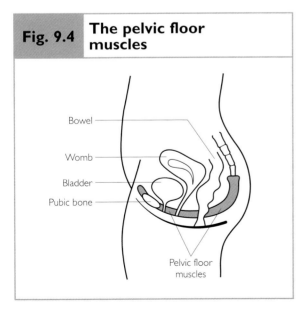

| Fig. 9.4 | **The pelvic floor muscles** |

Bowel
Womb
Bladder
Pubic bone
Pelvic floor muscles

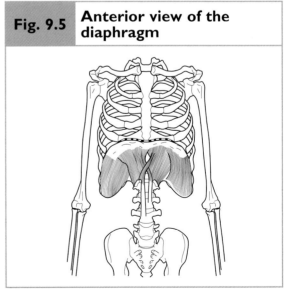

| Fig. 9.5 | **Anterior view of the diaphragm** |

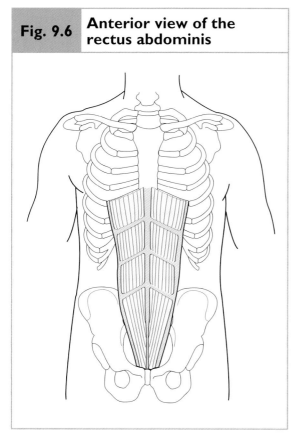

Fig. 9.6 Anterior view of the rectus abdominis

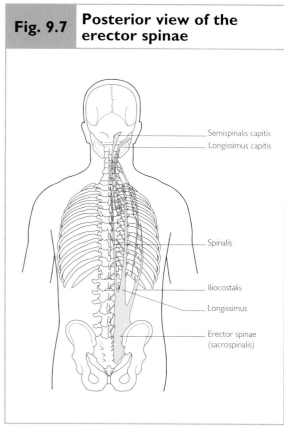

Fig. 9.7 Posterior view of the erector spinae

Semispinalis capitis
Longissimus capitis
Spinalis
Iliocostalis
Longissimus
Erector spinae (sacrospinalis)

Rectus abdominis

This muscle runs the length of the abdomen from the ribs down to the pubic bone and is held in place by fascia running horizontally across the muscle which gives it the appearance of having sections (see Fig 9.6).

Erector spinae

This essentially is a group of individual muscles that run either side of the spine from the sacrum and iliac crest to the base of the skull (see Fig 9.7).

External obliques

This superficial muscle lies almost at a vertical angle and runs from the surface of the lower 8 ribs down to the iliac crest (see Fig 9.8).

In order for the spine to remain protected at all times, it is essential that both the inner and outer units are working optimally. The ability of both units to function correctly is somewhat dependant on information relayed by the neuromuscular system. If this is not functioning optimally, the inner and outer units will not function optimally. Table 9.1 provides an overview of common local and global muscles and their characteristics.

TASK

Give a brief definition of the term 'core stabilisation' and describe the differences between stabilising and mobilising muscles in relation to inner and outer units.

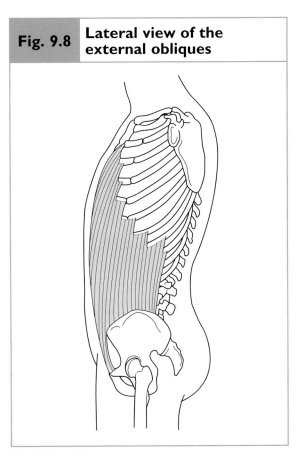

Fig. 9.8 **Lateral view of the external obliques**

Table 9.1	Common characteristics of local and global muscles	
	Local muscles (transversus abdominis, multifidus, pelvic floor, diaphragm, internal obliques)	Global muscles (rectus abdominis, external obliques, erector spinae)
Main fibre type	Slow-twitch	Fast-twitch
General task	Postural/endurance	Strength/explosive
Location	Deep	Superficial
Role	Stabilising	Mobilising
Common contraction	Isometric	Eccentric and concentric

Mechanisms of stabilisation

The mechanisms of stabilisation of the spine (core stability) are not fully understood, but it is thought that several systems, in conjunction with the ligaments of the spine, contribute to its overall stabilisation (although there is a body of evidence that disputes this). Systems such as *intra-abdominal pressure, thoraco-lumbar fascia gain* and the *hydraulic amplifier effect* are thought to provide enough spinal stabilisation for the body to carry out normal daily tasks. However, while the spine and its stabilisation systems are capable of protecting the spine under normal circumstances, an overload due to certain exercises, sport or poor posture can lead to a dysfunction in one or more of the systems, which could in turn lead to injury or postural problems (see Chapter 1 for common spinal injuries and postural problems).

Intra-abdominal pressure

In order to achieve an effective degree of core stability, the stabilising muscles of the inner unit must activate and contract together to help make the trunk more solid. This can be achieved in a number of ways, one of which is a process called intra-abdominal pressure.

The contents of the trunk area, including the stomach, intestines and various organs and fluid, are collectively termed the *abdominal ball* or *fluid ball*, which is cylinder-like in shape. When the core muscles contract, the walls of the abdominal ball are tightened and compressed. This creates an increase in pressure known as intra-abdominal pressure. This pushes against the spine and prevents it from making any excessive movements, and helps to keep the spine in the correct posture.

The example of an airbag inflated in a driver's seat can help to explain the process. It is difficult for the driver to move against

the airbag as the pressure resists his or her movement. The same principle applies with intra-abdominal pressure, where the abdominal ball resists the movements of the spine. In effect, this encourages the spine to move as a complete unit and prevents one part of the spine moving across another part of the spine, which could easily lead to injury.

The main muscles responsible for intra-abdominal pressure are: the transversus abdominis, the internal obliques and the multifidus muscles, which form the walls of the abdominal ball; the diaphragm, which forms the top of the abdominal ball; and the pelvic floor muscle, which forms the base of the abdominal ball. It is important that all of these muscles contract together so that the increase in pressure is evenly distributed along the spine. This requires an element of control, which is sometimes lost through lack of practice. It therefore requires a conscious effort and a lot of practice to achieve this contraction of the inner unit.

NEED TO KNOW

Researchers have found that in people with chronic low back pain the inner unit muscles do not function correctly. Dysfunction of the inner unit could be one of the causes of low back pain.

Thoraco-lumbar fascia gain

The *thoraco-lumbar fascia* is a sheet of connective tissue, almost tendon-like, that covers most of the muscles in the back and attaches to the spine, pelvis and sacrum. When the muscles of the inner unit are activated, tension is produced in the thoraco-lumbar fascia. It has been suggested that this tension creates an extension force on the spine (in other words, causes it to stiffen) and thus provides a degree of stabilisation that contributes to the overall stabilisation of the spine. The exact mechanism of thoraco-lumbar fascia gain is still under investigation and a topic of much debate.

Hydraulic amplifier effect

When the erector spinae muscles contract, the thoraco-lumbar fascia that surrounds these muscles resists their expansion. This resistance increases the strength of the erector spinae muscles by up to 30 per cent, and therefore it can be assumed that this effect contributes in some way to the stabilisation of the spine. Again, like thoraco-lumbar fascia gain, the hydraulic amplifier effect is currently being researched and the exact mechanisms are not yet fully understood.

TASK

Briefly explain the mechanisms that contribute to the overall stabilisation of the spine.

Neutral position or zone

The concept of the neutral position of the spine can be explained by thinking about the gears in a car. When a car is in neutral, there is no torque, or turning force on the gearbox. However, when the gears are engaged, considerable force is applied to make the car move. Similarly, when a normal functional spine is in its *neutral zone* (also known as *neutral*

spine), which is approximately midway between full posterior and anterior tilts of the pelvis, minimal force is placed on the spine and the structures that surround it (tendons, cartilage and ligaments). Any movement away from this position dramatically increases the stress placed on the surrounding tissues and hence the spine itself. Stabilisation control to maintain neutral spine is required when carrying out simple tasks such as sitting, as well as performing more complex tasks such as changing direction while running at speed, in order to prevent undue stress on the surrounding tissues that might eventually lead to injury. As mentioned above, this stabilisation control appears to be lacking in the majority of people who suffer from back pain and is thought to be one of the major causes of the back pain or injury responsible for the pain.

Awareness of the body and the position of its segments is a complex skill that requires practice – something that is made evident by the number of people who display poor posture. What appears to be neutral spine to an individual may not be considered neutral by the observer. Neutral spine can be found with the help of an observer by either standing or sitting on a stability ball and tilting the pelvis back and forward until the neutral position is found (see page 136). Tilting the pelvis forward (anterior tilt) increases the hollow in the lumbar spine area, whereas tilting the pelvis backward (posterior tilt) flattens the lumbar spine area. This method of finding neutral spine is not an exact science, but can be used to help the general population gain an awareness of posture. Instructors should be aware that if an individual has difficulty in achieving neutral zone then they may need to be referred to a person qualified to make a postural assessment.

Seated procedure for finding the neutral zone

Practitioner

1. Sit in an upright position on the stability ball with the knee joint just below the level of the hip joint and the feet shoulder-width apart.
2. Attempt to flatten the lower spine by pulling the crotch area up towards the chest (posterior tilt – see Fig. 9.9c).
3. Attempt to increase the hollow in the lower back by pulling the buttocks in a straight line towards the shoulder blades (anterior tilt – see Fig. 9.9a).
4. Repeat this movement several times at a slow, controlled pace.
5. Try to find the neutral position, after being informed of the correct position by the observer (see Fig. 9.9b).

See Fig. 9.9a–c.

Observer

1. Make sure that any movement occurs only in the lumbar spine; do not allow any movement at the shoulders or in the legs.
2. Watch for the full range of motion between the full anterior and the full posterior tilt.

Inform the practitioner when the pelvis is midway between these two points.

Fig. 9.9 **(a–c) Seated procedure for finding the neutral spine**

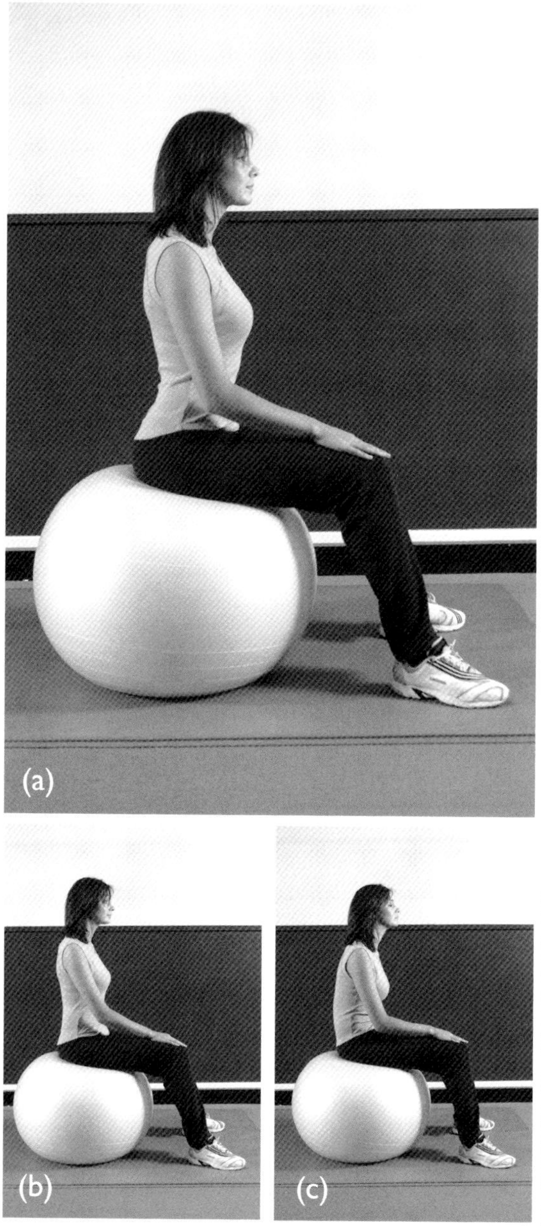

(a)

(b)

(c)

Standing procedure for finding the neutral zone

Practitioner

1. Stand in an upright position with the feet shoulder-width apart.
2. Attempt to flatten the lower spine by pulling the crotch area up towards the chest. (See Fig. 9.10a).
3. Attempt to increase the hollow in the lower back by pulling the buttocks in a straight line towards the shoulder blades. (See Fig. 9.10b).
4. Repeat this movement several times at a slow, controlled pace.
5. Try to find the neutral position after being informed of the correct position by the observer. (See Fig. 9.10c).

See Fig. 9.10a–c.

Observer

1. Make sure that any movement occurs only in the lumbar spine; do not allow any movement at the shoulders or in the legs.
2. Watch for the full range of motion between the full anterior and the full posterior tilt.
3. Inform the practitioner when the pelvis is midway between these two points.

NEED TO KNOW

To help prevent any unwanted movement, the observer can place both hands on the shoulders of the practitioner. The observer will feel any unwanted movement.

Fig. 9.10 **(a–c) Standing procedure for finding the neutral spine**

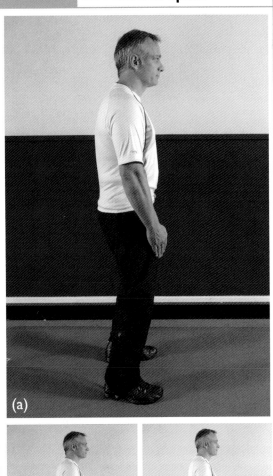

(a)

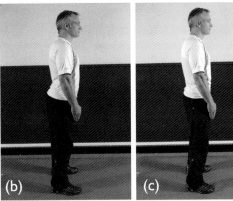

(b)   (c)

Contraction of the transversus abdominis (TA)

One of the mechanisms that can be used to achieve stabilisation of the spine is the principle known as the abdominal or *fluid ball* technique, as described on page 134. Through the contraction of certain stabilising muscles, pressure is placed upon the spine, which prevents unwanted movement and helps the spine to work as a unit. It would be almost impossible to consciously contract all of the muscles associated with stabilisation. When the transversus abdominis muscle is contracted either consciously or sub-consciously, the other muscles of the inner unit contract immediately afterwards.

Contraction of the stabilising muscles (inner unit) can be very difficult for several reasons. Many years of misuse, poor posture, overuse and weakness can result in a lack of subconscious activation of these muscles. As a result, it is common for exercises to be taught that are designed to improve subconscious activation of the inner unit muscles. One of the main difficulties associated with conscious activation is that many individuals try too hard, which usually results in the holding of breath and an increase in blood pressure. Research has suggested that only 30 per cent of the maximum contraction capability of the inner unit muscles is needed to create sufficient intra-abdominal pressure to stabilise the spine (Richardson et al., 2003).

Contraction of the transversus abdominis can be one of the most difficult conscious tasks for an individual to perform. However, for the contraction of the stabilising muscles to become subconscious (autonomous), it is essential to perform conscious practice of muscle contraction on a regular basis. The following method may be used to practise contraction of the transversus muscle, which will in turn activate the other stabilising muscles.

Conscious activation of the transversus abdominis

Body position

Lie with your back on the floor, knees bent and feet flat on the floor. Relax and try not to flatten the spine against the floor; instead, maintain a normal lumbar curve.

Hand position

Find a position two inches below the navel and two inches to either side of that position. Press in lightly on each side using the first two fingers of each hand. This should be the location of the transversus abdominis. Slide one hand under the natural curve of the lower spine so that you can feel any pressure changes from the body through the hand.

Initial contraction

Cough! As the transversus abdominis is one of the muscles responsible for the forced expiration of air during coughing, you should feel the contraction under your fingers (that is you should feel the muscle getting harder). The pressure on the hand under the lumbar spine should not change. Try to maintain constant pressure throughout the contraction.

Practice

The aim of the exercise is to try to replicate the contraction felt when coughing, without actually coughing. This can sometimes take a considerable amount of time to achieve, but once you can do it aim to contract at about 30 per cent of your maximum contraction capability.

Progression

Once you can contract the transversus abdominis, perform the same action without holding your breath or activating the rectus abdominis (a common mistake found in most people). You can place a hand just below the diaphragm to check for contraction of the rectus abdominis.

The lying method of contraction is suitable for initial purposes. Once individuals are capable of contracting their transversus abdominis, use the same method in a standing position. This makes it easier for individuals to perform the exercise on a daily basis.

The length of time, number of repetitions and frequency of practice of conscious contraction required to develop subconscious contraction control is different for every individual. It can be a lengthy process lasting up to several months, so it is recommended that conscious contraction practice be maintained for a period of no less than six months.

Typical core stability exercises

Once individuals are capable of contracting the transversus abdominis by conscious control, they can progress to other types of common stabilisation exercises. Individuals with no history of performing stabilisation exercises should initially be prescribed the most basic exercises and should only progress to more difficult exercises when they are comfortable with the previous level of stabilisation exercise.

The following core stability exercises should not be prescribed to clients who have back problems or who report pain when performing the exercises. Simple screening procedures (see Chapter 11) should be sufficient to identify individuals who should not be prescribed stabilisation exercises. The exercises might need to be deferred until the individual has been referred to a relevant professional and has been authorised to carry out an exercise programme.

Floor exercises

Kneeling abdominal hollow

See Fig. 9.11.

Starting position

1. Kneel on the floor with your shoulders directly above your hands and your hips directly above your knees.
2. Keep your head facing down towards the floor to prevent undue stress on the cervical spine.
3. Keep your knees shoulder-width apart. Check that your spine is in the neutral position.

Action

1. Consciously contract your transversus abdominis.
2. Breathe gently in and out, maintaining the contraction.
3. Breathe out and, before breathing in again, try to hollow your lower abdominals (imagine pulling your navel towards your spine).
4. Continuing to breathe normally, hold this position for a few seconds or until you are unable to hold it any more.
5. Repeat, trying to maintain normal breathing throughout.
6. Concentrate on maintaining the starting position during the course of the exercise.

Progressions

1. Try to perform the action without contracting the rectus abdominis.
2. Once you are comfortable with performing abdominal hollowing on all fours, try to perform the action in a standing position.
3. Try to contract the transversus abdominis without drawing in the lower abdominals. This is known as *abdominal bracing*.

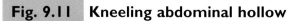

Fig. 9.11   Kneeling abdominal hollow

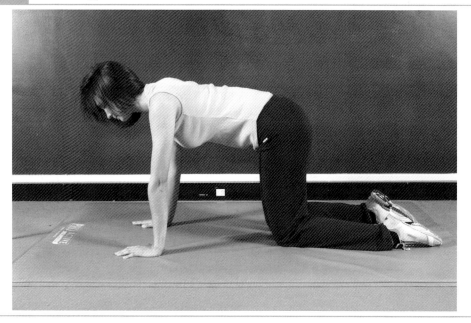

Supine foot slide

See Figs 9.12a and b.

Starting position

1. Lie on your back with your feet flat on the floor and your knees bent as much as is comfortably possible.
2. Place one arm down by your side and the other under the lumbar spine to check the pressure on your hand throughout the exercise.
3. Keep your knees shoulder-width apart. Check that your spine is in the neutral position.

Action

1. Consciously contract your transversus abdominis.
2. Breathe gently in and out.
3. Slowly slide one foot outwards along the floor until your leg is fully extended.
4. Return to the start position, trying to maintain normal breathing throughout.
5. Concentrate on keeping your spine in the neutral position during the exercise so that the pressure on your hand does not change.

Progressions

1. Once you are comfortable with the above action, try increasing the speed of the movement slightly.
2. Once you can perform the above exercise without a change in pressure on the hand under the lumbar spine, try sliding both legs out and back at the same time.

Fig. 9.12 **(a) and (b) Supine foot slide**

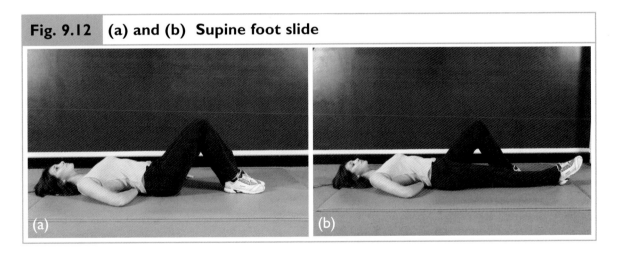

Pelvic tilts

See Figs 9.13a and b.

Starting position

1. Lie on your back with your feet flat on the floor and your knees bent as much as is comfortably possible.
2. Place your arms by your sides or across your abdomen.
3. Keep your knees shoulder-width apart. Check that your spine is in the neutral position.

Action

1. Consciously contract your transversus abdominis.
2. Breathe in and out gently.

3. Tilt your pelvis backward so that your lower back is flat on the floor (see Fig. 9.13b).
4. Return to the starting position, trying to maintain normal breathing throughout.

Progressions

1. Try performing the exercise while lifting one foot slightly off the floor.
2. As well as tilting the pelvis backward, try to tilt it forward so that your lumbar spine is more arched than normal.

Fig. 9.13   (a) and (b) Pelvic tilts

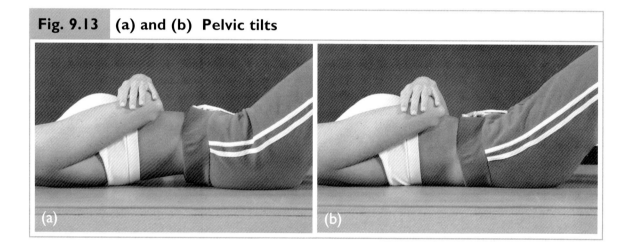

(a)   (b)

Side bridge

See Figs 9.14a and b.

Starting position

1. Lie on your side with your feet slightly apart to create a stable base.
2. Bend the arm nearest the floor at the elbow and rest it on the floor. This will provide support when you lift your upper body off the floor.
3. Put the opposite arm down by your side. Check that your spine is in the neutral position.
4. Keep your upper hip in line with your lower hip (see Fig. 9.14a).

Action

1. Consciously contract your transversus abdominis.

2. Breathe gently in and out.
3. Raise your lower hip off the floor so that your body forms a straight line (see Fig. 9.14b).
4. Hold this position until you start to feel muscle fatigue.
5. Try to maintain normal breathing throughout.
6. Concentrate on keeping your spine in the neutral position during the exercise.

Progression

Once you are comfortable with the above exercise, start with the hip in the raised position. Try to lower the hip nearest the floor towards the floor, then raise it to the start position again. Repeat.

Fig. 9.14 **(a) and (b) Side bridge**

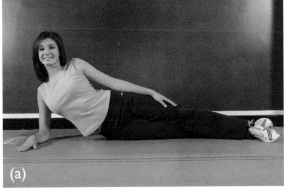
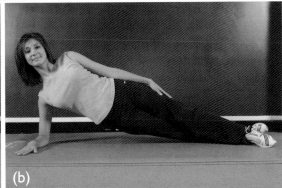

(a) (b)

Prone plank

See Figs 9.15a and b.

Starting position

1. Lie on your front with your feet slightly apart to create a stable base.
2. Place the forearms on the floor with the hands approximately at face level. This will provide support when you lift your body off the floor (see Fig. 9.15a).

Action

1. Consciously contract your transversus abdominis.
2. Breathe gently in and out.
3. Raise your body off the floor so that your body forms a straight line (see Fig. 9.15b).
4. Hold this position until you start to feel muscle fatigue.
5. Try to maintain normal breathing throughout.
6. Concentrate on keeping your spine in the neutral position during the exercise.

Progression

Once you are comfortable with the above exercise, try a plank position with straight arms.

Fig. 9.15 **(a) and (b) Prone plank**

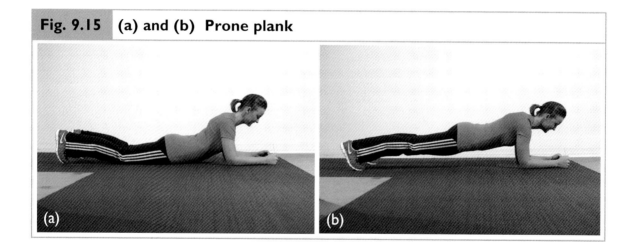

(a) (b)

Supine plank

See Figs 9.16a and b.

Starting position

1. Lie on your back with your feet slightly apart to create a stable base.
2. Bend the knees to approximately 90 degrees and keep the feet flat on the floor and the arms by your side. This will provide support when you lift your body off the floor (see Fig. 9.16a).

Action

1. Consciously contract your transversus abdominis.
2. Breathe gently in and out.
3. Raise your body off the floor so that your body forms a straight line (see Fig. 9.16b).
4. Hold this position until you start to feel muscle fatigue.

5. Try to maintain normal breathing throughout.
6. Concentrate on keeping your spine in the neutral position during the exercise.

Progression

Once you are comfortable with the above exercise, try keeping the plank position but raise one leg straight out in front. You could also try both positions with the arms across the chest.

Fig. 9.16 **(a) and (b) Supine plank**

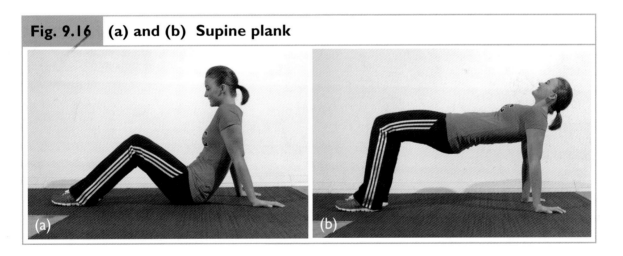

Stability ball exercises

Shoulder bridge

See Fig. 9.17.

Starting position

1. Sit upright on the ball.
2. Walk your feet forward and lean back at the same time until the ball is under your shoulder blades.
3. Lie face up with the ball under your shoulder blades.
4. Rest your head back onto the ball.
5. Keep your feet shoulder-width apart and your arms outstretched with the palms facing down.
6. Check that your spine is in the neutral position.
7. Keep a straight horizontal line through your shoulder, knee and hip joints.

Action

1. Consciously contract your transversus abdominis.
2. With your feet shoulder-width apart and your arms outstretched, gently roll a few inches to one side at the shoulders, then return to the start point.
3. Repeat, but roll to the opposite side.
4. Repeat this five times to each side.
5. Maintain normal breathing throughout.
6. Concentrate on maintaining the starting position during the exercise.

Safety point

Roll only as far as you feel in control of the movement. Use your hands to prevent yourself rolling if you go too far.

Fig. 9.17 **Shoulder bridge**

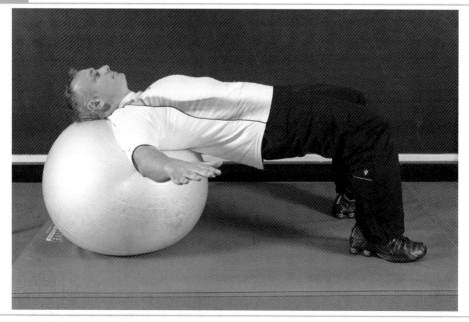

Foot bridge

See Fig. 9.18.

Starting position

1. Lie face up on the floor
2. Place the soles of your feet midway between the top and the side of the ball. Your knee joints should be at about 90 degrees at this point.
3. Keep your feet shoulder-width apart and your arms outstretched.
4. Raise your bottom off the floor until your spine is in the neutral position. Your legs tend to straighten at this point.
5. Only your shoulder blades, head and arms should be resting on the floor.

Action

1. Consciously contract your transversus abdominis.
2. With your feet shoulder-width apart and your arms outstretched, use your feet to roll the ball gently a few inches to one side, then return to the starting point.
3. Repeat, but roll to the opposite side.
4. Repeat five times to each side.
5. Maintain normal breathing throughout.
6. Concentrate on maintaining the starting position during the exercise.

Safety point

Roll only as far as you feel in control of the movement. If you lose control, adopt the starting position and repeat from the point at which you lost control.

Fig. 9.18 Foot bridge

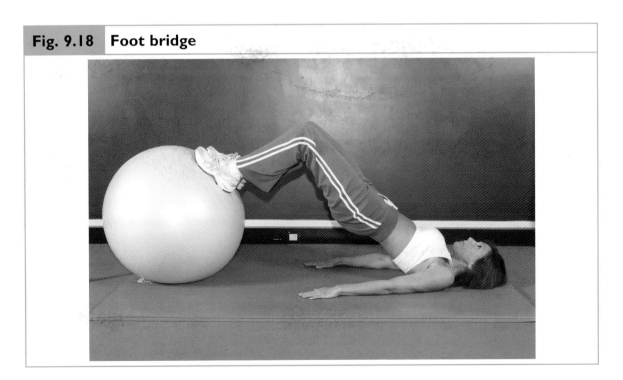

Straight-leg bridge

See Fig. 9.19.

Starting position

1. Lie face up on the floor.
2. Place the ball under your feet just below your heels.
3. Keep your feet shoulder-width apart and your arms outstretched.
4. Raise your bottom off the floor until your spine is in the neutral position.
5. There should be a straight line through the knee and hip joint.
6. Only your shoulder blades, head and arms should be resting on the floor.

Action

1. Consciously contract your transversus abdominis.
2. With your feet shoulder-width apart and your arms outstretched, use your feet to roll the ball gently a few inches to one side, then return to the starting point.
3. Repeat, but roll to the opposite side.
4. Repeat five times to each side.
5. Maintain normal breathing throughout.
6. Concentrate on maintaining the starting position during the exercise.

Safety point

Roll only as far as you feel in control of the movement. If you lose control, adopt the starting position and repeat from the point at which you lost control.

Fig. 9.19 **Straight-leg bridge**

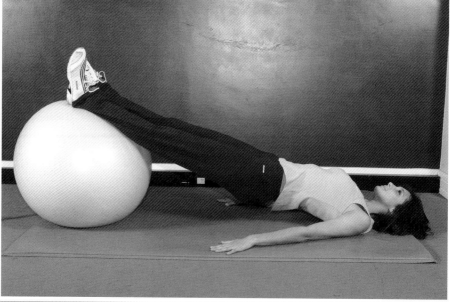

Front bridge

See Fig. 9.20.

Starting position

1. Kneel on the floor in front of the ball.
2. Lean forward over the ball so that your chest rests on the ball.
3. Roll over the top of the ball so that your forearms rest on the floor in front of the ball and your pelvis rests directly on top of the ball.
4. Check that your spine is in the neutral position.
5. Keep your neck in neutral by looking down at the floor.
6. Maintain a straight line through your knee, hip and shoulder joints.

Action

1. Consciously contract your transversus abdominis.
2. With your feet together and your forearms on the floor, gently roll the ball a few inches to one side and then return to the start point.
3. Repeat, but roll to the opposite side.
4. Repeat five times to each side.
5. Maintain normal breathing throughout.
6. Concentrate on maintaining the starting position during the exercise.

Safety point

Roll only as far as you feel in control of the movement. Put one foot on the floor if you feel you are about to lose control.

Fig. 9.20	**Front bridge**

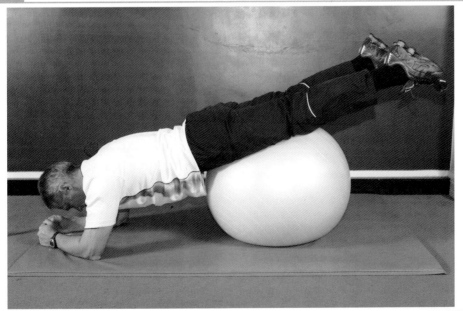

Ab burner

See Fig. 9.21.

Starting position

1. Kneel on the floor about 3 feet in front of the ball.
2. Lean forward over the ball so that your forearms rest on the ball.
3. Keep your knees shoulder-width apart.
4. Check that your spine is in the neutral position.
5. Keep your neck in neutral by looking at the floor in front of the ball.

Action

1. Consciously contract your transversus abdominis.
2. With your knees shoulder-width apart and your forearms on the ball, gently roll the ball a few inches to one side and then return to the start point.
3. Repeat, but roll to the opposite side.
4. Repeat five times to each side.
5. Maintain normal breathing throughout.
6. Concentrate on maintaining the starting position during the exercise.

Safety point

Roll only as far as you feel in control of the movement. Use your hands to prevent yourself rolling if you go too far.

Fig. 9.21   Ab burner

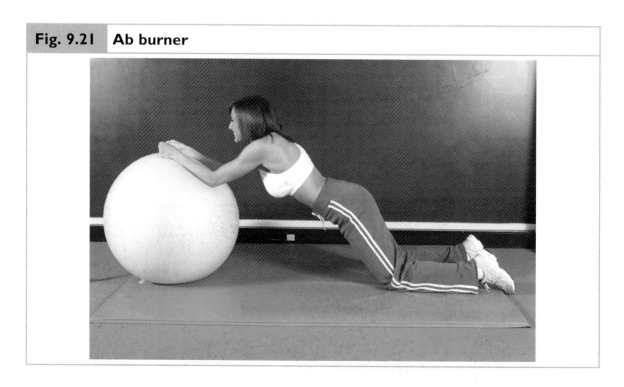

Floor push

See Figs 9.22a and b.

Starting position

1. Kneel on the floor about 3 feet in front of the ball.
2. Lean forward over the ball so that your hands rest on the ball.
3. Keep your knees shoulder-width apart.
4. Check that your spine is in the neutral position.
5. Keep your neck in neutral by looking at the floor in front of the ball.

Action

1. Consciously contract your transversus abdominis.
2. With the knees shoulder-width apart and your hands on the ball, gently lower your body until your chest comes to rest on the ball.
3. Gently raise your body back to the starting point by straightening your arms.
4. Repeat 10 times.
5. Maintain normal breathing throughout.
6. Concentrate on maintaining the starting position during the exercise.

Safety point

Lower your body only as far as feels comfortable.

Fig. 9.22 **(a) and (b) Floor push**

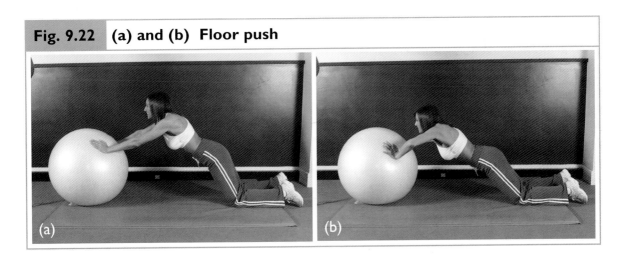

(a)   (b)

Exercise guidelines

In all new fitness or health programmes there is a period known as *habituation* during which the body, in particular the brain, becomes accustomed to the new form of exercise. When the brain becomes accustomed to the exercise, the body will adapt physically in order to accommodate the new level of exercise placed upon it. This period may last for several months. At this stage, the level of exercise can either be increased or maintained, depending on the individual's goals. Many factors influence the speed at which the body becomes accustomed to the new exercise regime or programme, such as frequency, duration, number of repetitions and ability level.

Frequency

Frequency is how often something occurs. In exercise, this is related to the number of times per week that the exercises are carried out. At the start of any new programme, at least two sessions per week are recommended in order for the body to adapt to cope with the regularity of the routine. Once the exercises have been carried out regularly for a period of a few weeks, the frequency of sessions can be reduced to once a week in order to maintain the adaptations that the body has made.

Duration

Duration relates to the amount of time spent on each exercise. The actual research carried out in this area is conflicting and there is no consensus as to the ideal duration of any one exercise. Every individual has a different objective and a different ability level, so it is impossible to recommend a duration period that would benefit all individuals equally. As a

general guide, however, start with an exercise duration of about 15 seconds. If the individual feels capable of increasing the duration, start by adding a period of five seconds to each exercise. If the individual feels that the duration for the exercise is too long, reduce the time of each exercise by five seconds until you reach a suitable duration.

NEED TO KNOW

Core stability training is effective when performed at a comfortable level; the 'no pain, no gain' saying is definitely not recommended in this case.

Repetitions

The number of repetitions simply refers to the number of times the exercise is repeated without a break. As core stability is not a strength issue, but relates to a learning process of the brain, the focus is on repeating the exercises at regular intervals to achieve this learning process as quickly as possible. Again, as research is unclear on the ideal number of repetitions, adjust the number of repetitions of each exercise to suit each individual's ability level. Once an individual becomes comfortable with this number of repetitions and feels able to perform more, increase the number until you reach a comfortable level.

NEED TO KNOW

If time is a concern, attempt as many repetitions as you are able. The old saying applies: 'anything is better than nothing'.

EXAMPLE QUESTIONS

9.1 Which of the following properties relates to stabilising muscles?
a) short-term, explosive, phasic, fast twitch
b) postural, endurance, phasic, fast twitch
c) short-term, endurance, phasic, slow twitch
d) postural, endurance, tonic, slow twitch

9.2 Which of the following properties relates to mobilising muscles?
a) short-term, explosive, phasic, slow twitch
b) postural, endurance, phasic, fast twitch
c) short-term, explosive, phasic, fast twitch
d) postural, endurance, tonic, slow twitch

9.3 Which of the following can be considered to be predominantly stabilising muscles for the core?
a) internal oblique, rectus abdominis, diaphragm
b) multifidus, transversus abdominis, pelvic floor
c) pelvic floor, external oblique, diaphragm
d) multifidus, erector spinae, internal oblique

9.4 Which of the following can be considered to be predominantly mobilising muscles for the core?
a) internal oblique, rectus abdominis, diaphragm
b) multifidus, transversus abdominis, pelvic floor
c) erector spinae, external oblique, rectus abdominus
d) multifidus, erector spinae, internal oblique

9.5 Which of the following can be considered to be a predominantly stabilising muscle for the hip joint?
a) internal obliques
b) gluteus maximus
c) transversus abdominis
d) gluteus medius

EXAMPLE QUESTIONS cont.

9.6 Which of the following can be considered to be predominantly a mobilising muscle for the hip joint?
a) internal obliques
b) gluteus maximus
c) transversus abdominis
d) gluteus medius

9.7 When local muscles contract to compress the 'fluid ball' in the abdomen it is known as what?
a) neutral spine or zone
b) intra-abdominal pressure
c) hydraulic amplifier effect
d) thoraco-lumbar fascia gain

9.8 An increase in the tension of the connective tissues in the spinal region is known as what?
a) neutral spine or zone
b) intra-abdominal pressure
c) fluid ball pressure
d) thoraco-lumbar fascia gain

9.9 Research has suggested that what percentage of maximum contraction is sufficient to create sufficient intra-abdominal pressure to stabilise the spine?
a) 70
b) 100
c) 50
d) 30

9.10 What best relates to the statement *'when there is minimal force placed on the spine and the structures that surround it such as tendons, cartilage and ligaments'*?
a) anterior pelvic tilt
b) neutral zone
c) intra-abdominal pressure
d) thoraco-lumbar fascia gain

EXAMPLE QUESTIONS cont.

9.11 True or False? Normal screening procedures should be carried out prior to prescribing core stabilisation exercises but those with back problems should be excluded.

True ☐   False ☐

9.12 The length of time, number of repetitions and frequency of practice of conscious contraction required to develop sub-conscious contraction control of the transversus abdominis can take up to how long?

a) a few hours
b) a few days
c) a few weeks
d) a few months

Further reading

Abrahams, P., Craven, J. and Lumley, J. (2011) *Illustrated Clinical Anatomy* (2nd ed.), Hodder Arnold

Handzel, T.M. (2003) 'Core training for improved performance', *NSCA's Performance Training Journal*, 2(6): 26–30

Liddle, D.S., Baxterb, D.G. and Graceya, J.H. (2009) 'Physiotherapists' use of advice and exercise for the management of chronic low back pain: A national survey', *Manual Therapy*, 14(2): 189–196

Marshall, P.W. and Murphy, B.A. (2005) 'Core stability exercises on and off a Swiss ball', *Archives of Physical Medicine and Rehabilitation*, 86(2): 242–249

Norris, C.M. (2001) *Abdominal Training* (2nd ed.), A&C Black

Norris, C.M. (2001) *Back Stability* (2nd ed.), Human Kinetics

Porter, S. (2002) *The Anatomy Workbook*, Butterworth Heinemann

Richardson, C., Jull, G., Hodges, P. andHides, J. (2003) *Therapeutic Exercise for Spinal Segmental Stabilization in Low Back Pain*, Churchill Livingstone

Ross, J.S. and Wilson, J.W. (2006) *Anatomy and Physiology in Health and Illness* (10th ed.), Churchill Livingstone

Sewell, D., Watkins, P. and Griffin, M. (2005) *Sport and Exercise Science: An Introduction*, Hodder Arnold

Tortora, G.J. and Grabowski, S.R. (2005) *Principles of Anatomy and Physiology* (11th ed.), Wiley

NOTES

COMPONENTS AND
PRINCIPLES OF FITNESS

10

OBJECTIVES

After completing this chapter, you will be able to:

1 Define the terms 'physical fitness', 'wellness' and 'health-related fitness'.

2 Define the term 'hypokinetic disease'.

3 List and describe the components of fitness.

4 State the ACSM guidelines relating to the components of fitness.

5 Describe how components of fitness can affect the body.

6 Explain the factors affecting physical fitness.

7 List and describe the principles of fitness.

8 List the main health risks associated with inactivity.

Level 2: Instructing Exercise and Fitness Knowledge

Basic Anatomy and Physiology

- The application of the principles and variables of fitness to the components of fitness.

- How to apply the principles and variables of fitness to a range of activities that will achieve various health benefits and the required fitness development.

Level 3: Instructing Physical Activity and Exercise Knowledge

Components of fitness

- Definitions of fitness:
  - Physical fitness
  - Health-related fitness
  - Wellness

- Components of fitness and how they can be assessed:
  - Aerobic capacity
  - Muscular strength
  - Muscular resistance

- • Flexibility
- • Body composition
- ■ Principles of fitness, including FITT, overload, specificity, reversibility
- ■ ACSM guidelines for developing each component of fitness
- ■ Methods of flexibility training (static, ballistic, dynamic, PNF, CRAC)

Introduction

This chapter deals with the components and principles of fitness in relation to guidelines within the National Occupational Standards framework for health and fitness, within which Level 2 and 3 instructors should be able to identify the components and principles of fitness and list the guidelines associated with these.

Later chapters in the book provide information regarding the practical application of theoretical knowledge, which, along with the content covered in this chapter, will provide you with the understanding and ability to design appropriate exercise programmes for apparently healthy individuals in line with current guidelines for exercise.

Definitions of fitness

There are many definitions and individual perceptions of 'fitness'. For some, fitness might include the ability to perform some activity at a competitive level, while to others it might be the ability to perform everyday tasks without undue stress and fatigue. Fitness might also include a health or wellness component, which can relate to the absence of disease.

Health-related physical fitness

The American College of Sports Medicine (ACSM) defines health-related physical fitness as

'an ability to perform daily activities with vigour and the demonstration of traits and capacities that are associated with a low risk of premature development of hypokinetic diseases.'

The closest translation for the word *hypokinetic* is 'low movement'. Hypokinetic diseases are associated with low levels of activity, such as heart disease, obesity and high blood pressure. For the purpose of this book, it is assumed that any prescribed exercise, regardless of the definition of fitness, will be beneficial in reducing the risk of hypokinetic disease.

Wellness

The ACSM definition of health-related physical fitness relates only to physical well-being, not to psychological well-being. However, there are many advocates of the notion that exercise can have a positive psychological effect, for example, promoting mental, social and emotional well-being. The World Health Organisation (WHO) promotes the idea of *wellness*, defining it as 'a state of complete physical, mental and social well-being, and not merely the absence of disease or infirmity'.

Physical fitness

Although the terms health-related physical fitness and wellness can be defined clearly, the most common anecdotal term used within the health and fitness industry is *fitness*. The ACSM distinguishes between health-related physical fitness and physical fitness, defining the latter as 'a set of attributes that relates to the ability to perform physical activity.'

Components of physical fitness

Fitness, or to be more precise physical fitness, can be divided into discreet components that can be trained or adapted individually. Depending on the type of training carried out, an individual can be classed as 'fit' in one or more of the individual components.

The ACSM lists the following components of health-related physical fitness: *cardiovascular endurance, muscular strength, muscular endurance, body composition* and *flexibility*. The components of physical fitness are the same, but also include *motor skills*, which comprise several sub-components. This book focuses on the components of health-related physical fitness.

Cardiovascular endurance

Cardiovascular endurance is the ability of the heart and lungs to deliver oxygen to the working muscles (sometimes known as *aerobic capacity*) and for the muscles to use this oxygen to generate work.

Measuring cardiovascular endurance

Cardiovascular endurance is often measured as *volume of oxygen (VO_2)*, with *VO_2max* being the maximum amount of oxygen that can be delivered to the working muscles. The units used to measure VO_2 are millilitres of oxygen per kilogram bodyweight per minute ($mlO_2.kg^{-1}.min^{-1}$).

How to improve cardiovascular endurance

The best types of exercise for improving cardiovascular endurance are those that involve

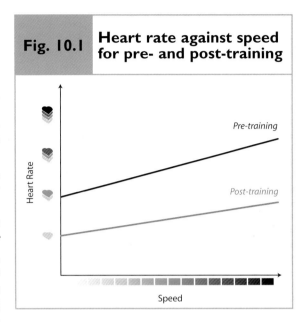

Fig. 10.1 **Heart rate against speed for pre- and post-training**

the use of large muscle groups over a prolonged period of time at an intensity that is classed as aerobic (for example, walking, hiking, running, stepping, swimming, cycling, dancing, skiing, skipping and so on). As the intensity of the exercise increases, the amount of oxygen required to cope with the demands made by the muscles increases; therefore, the heart rate increases in proportion. This increase in heart rate due to an increase in exercise intensity is known as a *linear relationship*. In other words, there is an equal increase in heart rate for an equal increase in intensity. Fig. 10.1 shows that after performing regular cardiovascular exercise for a period of time, the same intensity (speed) can usually be maintained with a lower heart rate.

FITT guidelines for cardiovascular training

It can be difficult to know the correct duration and intensity of exercise to recommend in order for your clients to achieve optimum benefits in terms of cardiovascular endurance.

Too little exercise might not have the desired effect, whereas too much might result in a condition known as *overtraining*, where damage to the body may occur in the form of an injury or a respiratory disease such as the common cold. For this reason, the ACSM has developed guidelines known as the *FITT principles*, which are recommended by governing bodies across Europe. FITT stands for *frequency*, *intensity*, *time* and *type*. Table 10.1 outlines the FITT guidelines for cardiovascular training.

Some clients may not be able to achieve 20 minutes of cardiovascular exercise or maintain intensities above 55 per cent of maximum heart rate. Therefore, the guidelines should be used to set targets for clients, rather than being absolute goals that clients must achieve. Any progressions should be limited to an increase of no more than 20 per cent of duration each week until clients can exercise at a moderate to vigorous intensity for 20–60 minutes. Increases in duration and frequency usually precede intensity increases.

Benefits of cardiovascular endurance

There are many benefits associated with an increase in cardiovascular endurance. One of the most important is a reduced risk in Coronary Artery Disease (CAD), and other benefits include:

- Reduced blood pressure
- Reduced body fat
- Lower heart rate for given intensity of exercise
- Increased exercise threshold for accumulation of blood lactate (the performer can exercise at a higher intensity before lactic acid builds up to the point at which intensity has to be reduced)
- Increase in HDL (good) cholesterol

Muscular strength

Muscular strength is the maximum amount of force that a muscle or muscle group can generate.

Measuring muscular strength

Both static and dynamic muscular strength can be measured. In static strength testing, machines called dynamometers measure how much force an individual can exert against it without any movement. In dynamic strength testing, an individual moves an external load (usually free weights or resistance machines). This is known as *1 repetition maximum* testing or *1RM* testing, where the maximum amount of weight that can be lifted once with good form is recorded. It is possible to predict 1RM from multiple RM testing, for example 6RM is the maximum amount of weight that can be lifted six times, which can then be used to predict IRM.

Table 10.1	FITT guidelines for cardiovascular training
Frequency	3–5 days per week
Intensity	55–90 per cent of maximum heart rate (RPE 12–16: see page 222)
Time	20–60 minutes continuous or intermittent aerobic exercise
Type	Involving large muscle mass; rhythmic; aerobic

How to improve muscular strength

Muscular strength can be developed through resistance training, including using machine and free weights, body weight and resistance bands. Developing muscular strength normally requires relatively high resistance (or weight) and few repetitions, and is usually associated with an increase in muscle size. Because of the intense nature of this type of training, it is common for individuals to experience pain or stiffness in the muscles that have been trained in the days following a training session. This sensation is known as delayed onset muscle soreness or DOMS.

Muscular endurance

Muscular endurance is the ability of a muscle or muscle group to perform repeated contractions against a resistance over a period of time, and is associated with resistance training using relatively low intensity and high repetitions. Hypertrophy is not usually associated with this type of training, although DOMS can be experienced if training is carried out to fatigue. Testing normally involves recording the maximum number of repetitions of a task, such as a push-up or sit-up that can be achieved.

Benefits of resistance training

There are many benefits of resistance training that vary slightly depending on the type of training. The benefits include the following:

- Increase in muscle mass, which increases resting metabolic rate
- Increase in bone mass
- Reduced risk of osteoporosis
- Increased glucose tolerance
- Increase in joint integrity
- Improved posture

- Reduction in back pain
- Reduced risk of hypertension
- Reduced risk of diabetes

The benefits of muscular endurance training are similar to those of muscular strength training, but with less emphasis on increased muscle mass and more emphasis on muscle tone. One of the long-term effects of resistance training is hypertrophy, or an increase in the size of the muscle being trained. This usually occurs after the first few weeks of training, as strength gains in the first few weeks are as a result of 'learning' mechanisms known as *neural* changes.

Delayed-onset muscle soreness (DOMS) can occur a day or two after a particularly intense training session. Light aerobic exercise following resistance training can reduce this effect.

FITT guidelines for resistance training

Table 10.2 outlines the FITT guidelines for resistance training.

Note: ACSM guidelines recommend a timing sequence of 3 seconds concentric and 3 seconds eccentric contraction for all resistance exercises that involve a full range of motion.

Volitional fatigue is the point at which the individual performing the exercise thinks that he or she can no longer carry on. This can be uncomfortable for the performer, so to encourage adherence to an exercise programme it is sensible to adopt a flexible approach to this guideline for individuals who are not familiar with exercising to fatigue levels.

Flexibility

Flexibility is the ability to move a joint through its complete range of motion.

Table 10.2	FITT principles for resistance training
Frequency	2–3 non-consecutive sessions per week
Intensity	1 set of 3–20 repetitions to volitional fatigue while maintaining good form (RPE 16–20)
Time	Enough to carry out 8–10 separate exercises for total body
Type	Body weight; machines; free weights; bands

Testing flexibility

Flexibility is joint specific in that an individual may be flexible in one joint and not in another. Therefore, there is no one test that is whole-body specific and all joints must be assessed individually using *goniometry*, where the angle of each joint is measured and compared against tables for normal ranges of motion. A common flexibility test used in the health and fitness industry is the 'sit and reach' test, where an individual sits with straight legs and reaches forward to record the distance reached with the fingertips. This measures only hamstring and upper back flexibility.

Benefits of flexibility

One of the main benefits of maintaining the range of motion within joints is that it allows individuals to carry out daily activities as long as possible throughout their lives. Although it is frequently recommended that stretching can help prevent injury, there is little evidence to support the notion: it has been shown that a high degree as well as a low degree of flexibility can increase injury risk. It is recommended that people with tight muscles would probably benefit most from static stretching whereas people who are naturally supple should not engage in more than light stretching. The most effective stretching occurs when the muscles are warm.

Types of stretching

There are many types of stretching exercise, including *static*, *dynamic*, *PNF* and *ballistic*. Below is a simple description of the common types of stretches.

Static stretching

A static stretch is held for a period of time at a point of mild tension. The point of tension is usually the point at which the stretch reflex is invoked. If the stretch is held for long enough, the tension usually subsides and the stretch can be taken further if required. If a partner or another group of muscles assists in the stretching process, it is known as an *active* stretch. If there is no assistance, it is a *passive* stretch. Research on the optimum time period for a stretch is vague, but guidelines relating to the recommended time period are shown in Table 10.3.

Dynamic stretching

A dynamic stretch refers to stretching in motion where an agonist muscle is contracted to stretch an antagonist muscle. This type of stretching is usually carried out in a slow and controlled manner in order to minimise the risk of injury and to mimic the types of movement that may be used in the exercises to follow.

Ballistic stretching

Ballistic stretches are bouncing movements caused by momentum or gravity. This type of stretching is usually carried out only by athletes who are familiar with this type of stretching: as there is little control of the movement, there is a greater risk of injury than with other types of stretching.

PNF stretching

PNF stands for proprioceptive neuromuscular facilitation. This is a type of partner-assisted stretching that is normally used for tight or injured muscles. This type of stretching requires training, so should be performed only by those who are qualified to do so. *CRAC* (Contraction Relax Antagonist Contract) is another form of this type of stretching.

Table 10.3 outlines the FITT guidelines for flexibility training.

Body composition

Body composition refers to the ratio of fat to lean tissue in an individual: in other words, how lean, overweight or obese a person is. Even though body composition is listed as a component of fitness, it is probably more accurate to associate it with an indication of health, as excess body fat is associated with hypertension, diabetes, stroke, coronary heart disease and hyperlipidaemia.

Body composition is also affected greatly by other components of fitness, such as cardiovascular and resistance training.

Measuring body composition

Body composition can be measured in many different ways, including BMI, using skinfolds, underwater weighing and electrical impedance methods. Some methods are more accurate than others. One of the easiest methods is BMI, or body mass index. Although this is not a direct measurement of body fat percentage, it does give an indication of overweight or obesity, which has been defined by the ACSM as the percentage of body fat at which an individual's risk of disease increases. BMI is calculated using the following equation:

$$BMI = \frac{Weight\ (kg)}{Height^2\ (m^2)}$$

Table 10.4 shows how BMI is used to classify body composition.

Although the causes of obesity can include hypothalmic, endocrine and genetic disorders, diet and physical inactivity are the prime factors. It is generally accepted and recommended by the ACSM that an increase in calorie expenditure and a decrease in calorie intake is the most effective long-term method for treating obesity:

Table 10.3	FITT guidelines for flexibility training
Frequency	Minimum 2–3 sessions per week; ideally 5–7 sessions per week
Intensity	To the end range of motion at a point of tightness, without pain
Time	15–30 seconds, 2–4 times per stretch
Type	Static, preceded by a warm-up

Table 10.4	BMI classifications
BMI	**Classification**
<25	Normal
25–30	Overweight
>30	Obese

between 150 and 400 Kcal of daily energy expenditure is recommended for weight-loss programmes.

Motor skills

Many sub-components are associated with motor skills, including speed, power, agility, co-ordination and balance. All of these areas can be improved with training.

Speed

Speed is the ability to move quickly from one point to another and can be improved through muscle co-ordination, efficient body movement, core strength and flexibility.

Power

Power is a combination of strength and speed and can be developed through plyometric and resistance training.

Agility

Agility is the ability to change direction at speed.

Balance

Balance is the ability to maintain equilibrium at all times. Proprioceptors in the body give information to the brain on the position of all limbs, as well as balance information from the inner ear and the eyes.

Co-ordination

Co-ordination is the ability to move the limbs precisely in a particular direction.

There are many theories regarding the storage of movement patterns, known as motor programmes. One theory proposed by Schmidt (1992) suggests that typical movements such as bending and squatting are stored with related information such as muscle timing and velocities. All other movements are just adaptations of these typical stored movements. For example, the movement sequence for a jump is similar to that of a squat because of the relationship of the body segments. A jump sequence, however, is entirely different from that of a leg press or leg extension. There are no recommended guidelines for motor skills in relation to FITT principles.

TASK

List and briefly describe the components of fitness and state the recommended guidelines related to each component.

Factors influencing physical fitness

When training for any of the components of fitness, various factors may influence the outcome of the type of training. These factors include *body type, gender, fitness level, lifestyle* and *age*.

Body type

The distribution of fibre type within muscles is determined at birth. A person with a higher percentage distribution of fast-twitch fibres will be more predisposed to strength-type events, whereas a person with a high percentage of slow-twitch fibres will be predisposed to endurance-type events.

There are three extreme classifications of body type that can be used to describe the overall shape of an individual: *endomorph, ectomorph* and *mesomorph* (see Table 10.5). It is common for individuals to be a combination of more than one type, so a grading system for each classification can be used.

Gender

Gender relates simply to either male or female. This has some implications on the components of fitness. For example, cardiovascular potential (VO_2max) is typically 15–30 per cent lower in females than in males. Men are also capable of greater muscle hypertrophy as a result of strength training, as they tend to have a greater proportion of fast-twitch fibres.

Table 10.5	Characteristics of different body types
Endomorph	• A pear-shaped body • A rounded head • Wide hips and shoulders • Wider front to back rather than side to side • A lot of fat on the body, upper arms and thighs
Ectomorph	• A high forehead • A receding chin • Narrow shoulders and hips • A narrow chest and abdomen • Thin arms and legs • Little muscle and fat
Mesomorph	• A wedge-shaped body • A cubical head • Wide, broad shoulders • Muscled arms and legs • Narrow hips • Narrow from front to back rather than side to side

Fitness

A less fit individual will initially make greater improvements in components of fitness than a fitter person. This should be taken into account when setting goals and targets with clients (see Chapter 12).

Lifestyle

There are many aspects of lifestyle that can affect components of fitness. One of the main aspects is psychological stress, which can have a detrimental effect on the way in which individuals train. Smoking and drinking alcohol can have a similar effect.

Age

Ageing can decrease the individual components of fitness, but with a regular training routine these diminishing effects can be minimised and in some cases reversed. For example, flexibility can very quickly be lost, but many older individuals retain flexibility by participating in exercises such as yoga.

TASK

Describe how various factors can influence physical fitness.

Principles of fitness

When designing any exercise programme it is important to remember certain fundamental factors that can have an affect on the outcome of the programme. These factors are called *principles of fitness*. These principles must be taken into account with all individuals in relation to the design of a training or exercise programme.

Specificity

The body can adapt to the demands of various types of exercise, and the type of adaptation that takes place is dependant on the muscle fibres involved and the types of exercise. For example, type 1 fibres will adapt to endurance training, while type 2 fibres will adapt to more intense strength training. The body will also adapt to the type (or specificity) of the training, For example, an individual who trains predominantly on a treadmill will become better at using the treadmill even though there will be a transfer of fitness to other types of cardio exercise.

Adaptation

This principle states that the adaptations derived from an exercise are specific to the exercise and to the muscles involved in that exercise. For example, runners show little improvement in the muscular endurance of their arm muscles, while cyclists show most of their muscular endurance improvement in their leg muscles. In order for adaptation in the body to occur, however, the body must be subjected to the exercise on a regular basis.

Overload

In order for an individual to adapt to a new demand or routine, overload must be achieved. Overload can be described as 'taking the body or system to a point just beyond what it is usually accustomed to' (ACSM, 2006). If any system within the body (a muscle or an organ) is made to work harder than it normally does on a regular basis, it will undergo certain physical changes to adapt to the new workload. It is important to remember that the body should be taken to a workload just beyond normal levels; if it is taken too far, injury may occur. There are many ways in which overload can be achieved within a programme in order to achieve adaptation. Lever length, speed, resistance and gravity are among many variables in which to progress a programme of exercise.

Progression

If the workload of a training programme is not progressed, the individual will not continue to adapt. Instead, once the body has adapted to the current workload, it will not attempt to adapt any further. In order to progress, the workload must be periodically changed once the body has become accustomed to the previous workload. The rate of progression is specific to each individual and can also be affected by various factors:

Fitness level

Less fit individuals will progress at a faster rate than fitter individuals.

Experience

An individual with past experience of certain exercises will progress at a faster rate than those with no experience.

Injury

An injury to a specific site can reverse any gains previously made at that site. It is important to remember that the rest of the body may be trained to prevent total body reversibility.

Environment

The nature of the environment can affect progression in several ways. For example, altitude training can have an effect on oxygen transport, while heat and cold can affect the rate of progression.

Regression (reversibility)

Just as the body can become stronger if the workload is increased, the body can become weaker over a period of time if the workload is reduced. It is possible for specific fitness components to diminish within two weeks of cessation of exercise. This principle is known as *regression*.

Individuality

As all individuals progress at different rates, it is important that frequency, intensity and duration of exercise are manipulated to suit the individual. In any health-related fitness programme, individuals should be encouraged to start slowly and begin at levels that can easily be maintained. Progression should then be encouraged when the individual feels that he or she can cope with the current workload and is able to progress.

Recovery time

It is often the case that the one thing missing from a progressive training programme is that of recovery time. It is obvious that rest is just as important in any exercise programme as active recovery periods. Instructors should constantly monitor individuals for signs of exhaustion and over-training, such as a drop in performance, increase in resting heart rate and regular illness. Recovery of the muscular, cardiovascular and neural systems depend on many factors, such as the intensity of the training session, individual fitness levels, age, psychological factors and dietary interventions. As a very general guideline, individuals should be given a 24–48-hour recovery period following a bout of exercise. This can be split, however, so that training can take place each day. With resistance training, for example, daily sessions could take place but different muscle groups could be targeted on different days to allow recovery.

TASK

List and briefly explain the principles used in prescribing exercise.

Health risks of inactivity

The benefits of undertaking regular physical activity are well documented throughout this book. However, it should be noted that there are many health risks associated with inactivity. In 2002, a report from the World Health Organization (WHO) stated that physical inactivity (less than 2.5 hours per week moderate intensity activity or 1 hour per week of vigorous activity) is one of the ten leading causes of death in developed countries, resulting in more than 1.9 million deaths worldwide per year. There are many published reports that discuss the range of health risks associated with physical inactivity (or being sedentary as it is usually referred to) of which table 10.6 shows common examples. For information purposes, the Department of Health (2004) classifies active people as having an energy expenditure of 500–1,000Kcals per week which is about 6 to 12 miles of walking (roughly 10,000 to 20,000 steps per week) for an average-weight individual.

Table 10.6	Health risks of inactivity
Condition	**Incidence and effect of physical activity (PA)**
Coronary heart disease (CHD)	In the UK about 38% of CHD related deaths are as a result of PA or sedentary lifestyles. Inactive people are almost twice as likely to have a heart attack as active people (Department of Health 2000).
Stroke	According to the British Heart Foundation (2005), stroke accounts for about 9% of all deaths in men and about 13% of all deaths in women in the UK. Research suggests that moderately active people are less likely to have a stroke or die of stroke-related causes than people with low activity levels.
Certain cancers	It is estimated that more than 7000 women in England alone died prematurely from breast cancer in the year 2000. It has been widely reported that regular PA is associated with a decreased risk of developing colon cancer by up to 50%.
Diabetes	About 1.5 million people in the UK have been diagnosed with Type 2 diabetes. Regular PA can lower the risk of developing non-insulin dependent diabetes mellitus by as much as 50% (NHS 2009).
Hypertension	High blood pressure affects more than 16 million people in the UK and is the direct cause of about half of all strokes and heart attacks in the country. Regular PA prevents or delays the development of high blood pressure (Health Survey for England 2007).
Osteoporosis	According to Van Staa (2001), in the UK about 1 in 2 women and 1 in 5 men over the age of 50 will sustain a spine, hip or wrist fracture mainly as a result of osteoporosis. Strength training in older women has been shown to reduce the risk of hip fracture by up to 50%.
Obesity	In England in 2007 about 65% of men and 56% of women were overweight (this is including those that are obese). Regular PA can reduce the risk of becoming obese by as much as 50% compared to people with sedentary lifestyles (NHS 2009).
Anxiety and depression	Regular PA appears to: relieve symptoms of depression and anxiety, improve mood and self-esteem and protect against the development of mild forms of depression (Kugler 1994 and Boutcher 2000).
Osteoarthritis	According to the Arthritis Research Campaign in 2002, arthritis (in all forms) affects about 7 million people (more than 10%) in the UK at any one time. Research has shown that an absence of stress on the joints can increase the risk of osteoarthritis (as can an excess of stress).

EXAMPLE QUESTIONS

10.1 The ACSM define what as *'an ability to perform daily activities with vigour and the demonstration of traits and capacities that are associated with a low risk of premature development of hypokinetic diseases'*?

a) wellness
b) physical fitness
c) health related physical fitness
d) mental health

10.2 The World Health Organisation defines what as *'a state of complete physical, mental and social well-being and not merely the absence of disease or infirmity'*?

a) wellness
b) physical fitness
c) health related fitness
d) mental health

10.3 Cardiovascular endurance is also known as what?

a) anaerobic capacity
b) aerobic capacity
c) ventilatory capacity
d) respiratory capacity

10.4 $mlO_2.kg^{-1}min^{-1}$ is a measurement of what?

a) anaerobic capacity
b) lactate threshold
c) VO_2max
d) OBLA

10.5 What are the benefits of regular cardiovascular training?

a) increased HDL, increased exercise threshold, decreased heart rate for given intensity
b) decreased HDL, increased exercise threshold, decreased heart rate for given intensity
c) increased HDL, increased exercise threshold, increased heart rate for given intensity
d) increased HDL, decreased exercise threshold, decreased heart rate for given intensity

EXAMPLE QUESTIONS cont.

10.6 What is the term used to define an increase in muscle cross-section?
a) DOMS
b) atrophy
c) hypertrophy
d) tone

10.7 What is the term used to define a decrease in muscle cross-section?
a) DOMS
b) atrophy
c) hypertrophy
d) tone

10.8 What are the benefits of regular resistance training?
a) increased glucose tolerance, increased bone mass, increased resting metabolic rate
b) increased glucose tolerance, increased bone mass, decreased resting metabolic rate
c) decreased glucose tolerance, increased bone mass, increased resting metabolic rate
d) increased glucose tolerance, decreased bone mass, increased resting metabolic rate

10.9 Strength gains in the first few weeks of a resistance training programme are usually due to what?
a) hormonal changes
b) muscular atrophy
c) hypertrophy changes
d) neural changes

10.10 What type of stretching involves the contraction of the agonist to elicit a stretch in the antagonist?
a) static
b) dynamic
c) ballistic
d) PNF

EXAMPLE QUESTIONS cont.

10.11 Which of the following formulae can be used to calculate BMI?
- **a)** weight^2 / height
- **b)** weight / height^2
- **c)** height / weight^2
- **d)** height^2 / weight

10.12 In relation to BMI, what figure is classed as obese?
- **a)** over 25
- **b)** over 30
- **c)** over 20
- **d)** over 15

Further reading

American College of Sports Medicine (2009) *ACSM Guidelines to Exercise Testing and Prescription* (8th ed.), Lippincott, Williams and Wilkins

Baechle, R.T. (2008) *Essentials of Strength Training and Conditioning* (3rd ed.), Human Kinetics

Bird, S.P., Tarpenning, K.M. and Marino, F.E. (2005) 'Designing resistance training programmes to enhance muscular fitness: a review of the acute programme variables', *Sports Medicine*, 35: 841–851

Bompa, T.O. and Haff, G.G. (1999) *Periodisation Theory and Methodology of Training* (5th ed.), Human Kinetics

Bouchard, C., Shepard, R. and Stephens, T. (1994) *Physical Activity, Fitness and Health*, Human Kinetics

Boutcher, S.H. (2000) 'Cognitive performance, fitness and ageing', in Biddle, S.J.H., Fox, K.R., & Boutcher, S.H., *Physical Activity and Psychological Well-Being*, Routledge, 118–129

British Heart Foundation Health Promotion Research Group (2005) *Coronary Heart Disease Statistics*, University of Oxford: Department of Public Health

Department of Health (2000) *Coronary Heart Disease: National Service Framework for coronary heart disease – Modern standards and service models*, DoH

Department of Health (2004) *At Least 5 a Week: Evidence on the impact of physical activity and its relationship to health*, DoH

Department of Health, Health Survey for England (2007) *Healthy Lifestyles: Knowledge, attitudes and behaviour*, NHS Information Centre for Health and Social Care

Fleck, S.J. and Kraemer, W.J. (2003) *Designing Resistance Training Programs* (3rd ed.), Human Kinetics

Howley, E.T. and Franks, B.D. (2003) *Health Fitness Instructor's Handbook* (4th ed.), Human Kinetics

Kugler, J., Seelbach, H. and Kruskemper, G.M. (1994) 'Effects of rehabilitation exercise programmes on anxiety and depression in coronary patients: a meta-analysis', *British Journal of Clinical Psychology*, 33: 401–410

Marieb, E.N. (2009) *Human Anatomy and Physiology* (8th ed.), Benjamin Cummings Publishing Company Inc.

McArdle, W.D., Katch, F.I. and Katch, V.L. (2007) *Exercise Physiology* (6th ed.), Lippincott, Williams & Wilkins

NHS information Centre, Lifestyle Statistics (2009) *Statistics on Obesity, Physical Activity and Diet: England, February 2009*, NHS Information Centre for Health and Social Care

Plisk, S.S. and Stone, M.H. (2003) 'Periodization strategies', *Strength and Conditioning Journal*, 25: 19–37

Ross, J.S. and Wilson, J.W. (2006) *Anatomy and Physiology in Health and Illness* (10th ed.), Churchill Livingstone

Sewell, D., Watkins, P. and Griffin, M. (2005) *Sport and Exercise Science: An Introduction*, Hodder Arnold

Schmidt, R.A. (2003) 'Motor schema theory after 27 years: reflections and implications for a new theory', *Research Quarterly for Exercise and Sport*, 74(4): 366–375

Tortora, G.J. and Grabowski, S.R. (2005) *Principles of Anatomy and Physiology* (11th ed.), Wiley

Van Staa, T.P., Dennison, E.M., Leufkens, H.G. and Cooper, C. (2001) 'Epidemiology of fractures in England and Wales', *Bone*, 29: 517–522

Wilmore, J.H. and Costhill, D.L. (2011) *Physiology of Sport and Exercise* (5th ed.), Human Kinetics

World Health Organization (2002) *The World Health Report 2002: Reducing risks, promoting healthy life*, WHO Press

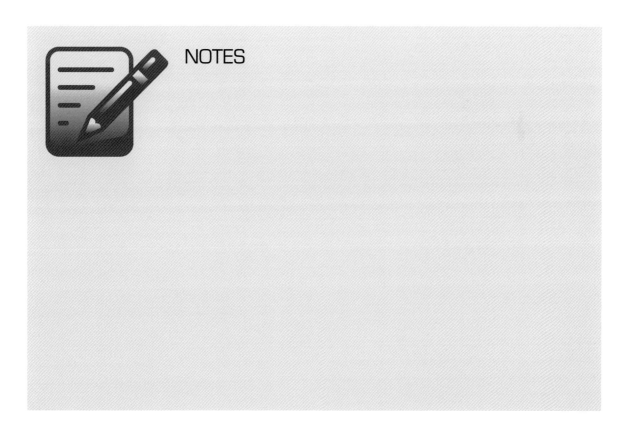

NOTES

NOTES

PRACTICAL APPLICATION OF HEALTH AND FITNESS

PART TWO

Part 2 looks at practical methods of applying the theory covered in Part 1. Each chapter provides example questions that are typical of industry-standard Level 2 and 3 questions provided by accredited centres for the delivery of recognised qualifications. There is also a list of recommended reading for each chapter, should you wish to gain more in-depth knowledge of a particular subject area.

SCREENING FOR EXERCISE
AND SAFETY ISSUES

OBJECTIVES

After completing this chapter, you will be able to:

1 Define the term 'screening' in relation to the health and fitness industry.

2 List and describe the different types of screening questionnaire available for the health and fitness industry.

3 Explain the term 'risk stratification' and list the coronary artery risk factors identified by the American College of Sports Medicine.

4 Briefly outline the areas of the Health and Safety at Work Act 1974 relating to the health and fitness industry.

5 Describe general issues relating to facility equipment management.

6 Describe procedures of risk assessment relating to hazards prior to exercise sessions.

7 Explain the procedure for dealing with an emergency situation during an exercise session.

8 Briefly outline the Health and Safety (First Aid) Regulations 1981 pertaining to the health and fitness industry.

9 Briefly discuss methods of reporting accidents and incidents.

10 Briefly discuss issues relating to child protection and how to seek further information.

Level 2: Instructing Exercise and Fitness Knowledge

Basic Anatomy and Physiology

- The importance of careful and thorough planning and preparation for sessions.

- The requirements for health and safety that are relevant to the activities you are planning, for example: factors that affect group/individual working space, your organisation's health and safety policies and procedures, the Health and Safety at Work Act.

- The factors that affect the ability to exercise; the screening process, including primary and secondary risk factors of coronary heart disease.

- The Exercise and Fitness Code of Ethical Practice.

- Reasons for temporary deferral of exercise; referral; informed consent.

- The emergency procedures of the facility/organisation.

- The Pre-Activity Readiness Questionnaire (PAR-Q) and how to record information on it.

- How to identify and agree objectives for the session based upon collected information.

- Manufacturers' and organisations' guidelines for replacement of equipment.

- The safe storage of free-weight equipment.

- What to look for when checking equipment.

- The health and environmental factors that can influence safety; factors that affect group/individual working space.

Level 3: Instructing Physical Activity and Exercise Knowledge

Components of Fitness
- Coronary heart disease risk factors

Introduction

This chapter deals with various screening methods used within the health and fitness industry, as well as looking at safety issues in relation to guidelines within the National Occupational Standards framework for health and fitness. Level 2 and 3 instructors should be able to identify safety issues and describe methods of screening and the guidelines associated with these.

Later chapters in the book provide the knowledge required in relation to programme design, which, along with the content covered in this chapter, will provide you with the understanding and ability to design appropriate exercise programmes for apparently healthy individuals, in line with current guidelines for exercise.

Screening for exercise

One of the most important roles of a health and fitness instructor is to help individuals determine their current health and fitness status prior to undertaking a programme of exercise. Not only can this aid in planning and designing a safe and effective programme, but also in identifying any professional guidance that may be needed before the individual undertakes the programme. If any condition is identified which places the individual in a *special population* category (see *Teaching Exercise to Special Populations* by Morc Coulson) and that the instructor is not qualified to deal with, they should inform the individual that this is the case and that they may only have a basic knowledge of the condition.

The process of determining the health and fitness status of an individual is known as *health screening*, normally shortened to *screening*. In a health and fitness environment, two methods of screening are available to the instructor. One method involves the use of pre-exercise questionnaires, of which there are many types, and the other involves verbal methods.

Pre-exercise questionnaires

Health screening questionnaires

Many types of pre-exercise health questionnaires are available, the most common in the health and fitness industry being the *Physical Activity Readiness Questionnaire*, or *PAR-Q* (see Fig. 11.1 for an example). Developed by the Canadian Society for Exercise Physiology, the PAR-Q is a short questionnaire that can help to identify possible symptoms of cardiovascular, pulmonary and metabolic disease, as well as other conditions that might be aggravated by exercise. The form is self-explanatory and brief: if any conditions are identified, the form advises the individual to seek medical approval prior to undertaking a programme of exercise. If no conditions are identified, the form encourages a programme of light to moderate exercise to be undertaken at an intensity relevant to the current fitness level of the individual.

PAR-Q forms should be given out to all individuals and completed prior to the start of an exercise programme. The form should then be interpreted by a suitably qualified professional and dealt with in a confidential manner. If the instructor feels that the form reveals anything that is beyond the capacity of their training or experience, they should refer the case to a suitably qualified colleague or supervisor. It should also be noted that PAR-Qs are normally only valid for a 12-month period.

Fig. 11.1	**Example of a PAR-Q**

PAR-Q and You

Please read the following questions and answer each one honestly.   Yes   No

1. Has your doctor ever said that you have a heart condition and that you should
   only do physical activity recommended by a doctor?   —   —

2. Do you feel pain in your chest when you do physical activity?   —   —

3. In the past month, have you had chest pain while you were not doing physical activity?   —   —

4. Do you lose your balance because of dizziness or do you ever lose consciousness?   —   —

5. Do you have a bone or joint problem that could be made worse by physical activity?   —   —

6. Is your doctor currently prescribing drugs for your blood pressure or heart condition?   —   —

7. Do you know of any other reason why you should *not* do physical activity?   —   —

If you answered YES to one or more questions:
Talk to your doctor **BEFORE** you become more physically active or have a fitness appraisal. Discuss with your doctor which kinds of activities you wish to participate in.

If you answered NO to all questions:
You can be reasonably sure that you can:

- Start becoming much more physically active. Start slowly and build up gradually.
- Take part in a fitness appraisal. This is a good way to determine your basic fitness level. It is recommended that you have your blood pressure evaluated.

Fig. 11.1	Example of a PAR-Q cont.

However, delay becoming active if:

- You are not feeling well because of temporary illness such as a cold or 'flu.
- You are or may be pregnant: talk to your doctor first.

Please note: *If your health changes so that you then answer YES to any of the above questions, tell your fitness or health professional. Ask whether you should change your physical activity plan.*

'I have read, understood and completed this questionnaire. Any questions I had were answered to my full satisfaction.'

Name: _____

Signature: _____

Date: _____

Signature of witness: _____

Signature of parent/guardian: _____

Note: This physical activity clearance is valid for a maximum of 12 months from the date it is completed, and becomes invalid if your condition changes so that you would answer YES to any of the seven questions.

Source: Physical Activity Readiness Questionnaire (PAR-Q) 2002. Reprinted with permission from the Canadian Society for Exercise Physiology.

Physical activity screening questionnaires

Prior to designing a programme of exercise for an individual, it is recommended that previous and current client fitness levels are established. One of the methods commonly employed within the health and fitness industry is a *physical activity screening questionnaire*, which is often used to ensure the exercise programme is at the optimum level for the client. However, a fitness questionnaire is not a replacement for the PAR-Q, but rather a supplement to it.

There is no accepted standard of fitness questionnaire available and many different types are used within the health and fitness industry. Typical questionnaires include the following questions:

1. Do you currently participate in any form of exercise?
2. How often do you participate in exercise?
3. What types of exercise do you currently participate in?
4. How long do you normally exercise for during each session?
5. Would you class your exercise as moderate or vigorous?
6. Can you walk briskly for 30 minutes without fatigue?
7. Can you jog for 20 minutes without fatigue?
8. What types of exercises do you enjoy doing?
9. What types of exercise do you not like doing?
10. If you do not currently exercise, when was the last time you participated in regular exercise?
11. How often did you participate in regular exercise and what type of exercise was it?

As with all information of a personal nature, the physical activity screening questionnaire must be treated confidentially. Confidentiality and other such values are explained in more detail within a set of standards known as the Code of Ethics. This applies to instructors within the health and fitness industry and constitutes a set of guidelines within which to work. For more details visit www.skillsactive.co.uk.

Lifestyle questionnaires

Lifestyle questionnaires are also commonly used in the health and fitness industry to elicit information about diet, exercise and activities regarded as *lifestyle activities*, such as walking, housework and gardening. Lifestyle activities have been shown to have numerous health benefits and can be integrated into a typical daily lifestyle for most individuals, and these types of questionnaires can help instructors to identify areas of lifestyle that could be improved and could be incorporated into an overall programme of exercise. It must be stressed, however, that recommendations relating to diet are limited by national occupational standards and advice beyond this should only be given by those who are qualified in this area.

As with physical activity screening questionnaires, lifestyle questionnaires are not a replacement for the PAR-Q but a supplement to it. Many lifestyle questionnaires are in use in the health and fitness industry, but typical questionnaires include the following questions:

1. Do you currently smoke and, if so, how much?
2. Do you drink alcohol and, if so, how much on average each week?
3. Do you work at a desk each day?
4. How do you travel to work?
5. What do you do at break times?
6. Are there any stairs at your place of work?
7. What is your typical daily routine?
8. How far do you walk on a typical day?
9. Would you consider yourself to have a healthy diet?
10. Do you snack between meals?
11. When do you have your last meal of the day?

Note: With all pre-exercise questionnaires, the instructor must respect the confidentiality of all written material relating to client information by ensuring safe storage and private access.

Verbal screening

In addition to the PAR-Q screening form, instructors can screen clients verbally prior to an exercise session. A certain amount of time may have elapsed between a client completing a PAR-Q and actually beginning a programme of exercise. Within this period of time injuries may have occurred, so individuals should be asked if they know of any reason why they should not exercise or if they have any current injury that could prevent them from exercising. In certain facilities, it is also possible for members to access studio classes without going through the screening process. For this reason, when supervising a one-to-one or group exercise session, it is advisable to carry out verbal screening prior to the start of the session.

It is at the instructor's discretion to decide whether any response warrants medical referral. All GP surgeries have their own procedure for exercise referral, so it is important to be aware of the procedures employed at geographically relevant surgeries. Verbal screening is also confidential, therefore discretion must be used in a group exercise situation.

Note: Some health and fitness facilities use an informed consent form that individuals agree to and sign before undertaking an exercise programme. These forms state the benefits and risks associated with exercise and are intended as a precaution against liability.

TASK

List the types of screening available to instructors and describe the benefits of each.

Risk stratification

Although the PAR-Q screening process is considered an acceptable level of screening within the health and fitness industry, many other more in-depth health screening questionnaires can be used. These questionnaires can provide a more detailed medical and lifestyle history.

One such questionnaire is the AHA/ACSM Health/Fitness Facility Pre-participation Screening Questionnaire (see Fig. 11.2), which can identify a broad range of diseases that can be aggravated by exercise. It can also help to identify certain conditions that have been shown to increase the risk of heart disease, known as coronary artery disease risk factors. The American College of Sports Medicine identifies the following as coronary artery disease risk factors:

1. **Family history:** myocardial infarction (MI) or sudden death before age 55 in father, brother or son; before age 65 in mother, sister or daughter.
2. **Smoking:** current smoker or quit within previous six months.
3. **Hypertension:** systolic blood pressure of 140mmhg or above, or diastolic of 90mmhg or above, on at least two occasions.
4. **Dyslipidaemia:** total serum cholesterol of more than 5.2mmol/L, or LDL more than 3.4mmol/L, or HDL less than 1.03mmol/L.
5. **Obesity:** BMI of $30kg/m^2$ or above.
6. **Sedentary lifestyle:** not participating in regular exercise.
7. **Impaired fasting glucose:** 100mg/dL or more.

Fig. 11.2	Example of a risk stratification questionnaire	
Mark all true statements		

History – You have had:

____ a heart attack
____ heart surgery
____ cardiac catheterisation
____ coronary angioplasty
____ a pacemaker
____ defibrillator
____ heart valve disease
____ heart failure
____ a heart transplant
____ heart disease

Symptoms – You experience:

____ chest pain with exertion
____ unreasonable breathlessness
____ dizziness or fainting
____ heart medication

Other issues:

____ you have diabetes
____ you have asthma or COPD
____ you get a burning sensation in the legs when walking short distances
____ you have musculoskeletal problems that limit physical activity
____ you have concerns about exercise safety
____ you take prescribed drugs
____ you are pregnant

Risk factors:

____ you are a male over 45 years old
____ you are female over 55 years old
____ you smoke or have quit within the last six months
____ your blood pressure is above 140/90 mmhg
____ your total cholesterol is above 5.2 mmol/L
____ you have heart attack or sudden death in the family (male before 55 years, female before 65 years)
____ you are sedentary
____ you are classed as obese

> If you marked any of the statements in this section as true, consult your GP before taking part in an exercise programme.

____ none of the above	You can exercise.

Adapted from the AHA/ACSM Health/Fitness Facility

It should be noted that family history is classed as an unmodifiable risk factor in that nothing can be done about it in terms of exercise, whereas the others are classed as modifiable risk factors in that exercise can have an impact on them.

Pre-participation screening

Once the individual has completed the questionnaire, they can be classified into one of three categories: *low risk* (or apparently healthy), *moderate risk* and *high risk* (see Table 11.1). This process is known as *risk stratification.*

The ACSM states that individuals who have two or more risk factors, men who are 45 or older and women who are 55 or older have a moderate risk factor. It is not recommended that individuals in this category be prescribed any vigorous exercise unless medical approval is given. Individuals in the high-risk category should not be allowed to exercise unless supervised by a qualified person.

NEED TO KNOW

If an individual has an HDL cholesterol reading greater than 1.6mmol/L, subtract one risk factor from their total.

Health and safety issues

It is important for health and fitness instructors to be aware that they need to address many health and safety issues due to the emerging litigational environment that they work in and, more importantly, for the safety of their clients. The main areas for concern are health and safety at work, equipment management, risk assessment, emergency first aid, potential accidents/incidents and child protection.

Health and safety at work

As in any environment, health and safety is an issue in any facility in which exercise is undertaken. The Health and Safety at Work Act (HSWA) 1974 outlines the role of the instructor (as well as those appointed persons for all areas of health and safety) in relation to prevention of accidents and, although the HSWA is an extensive document, a selection of the roles relevant to the health and fitness instructor are as follows:

1. Take responsible care for their own safety and that of others.
2. Co-operate with employers in matters of safety.
3. Do not interfere with or misuse anything provided for safety.

Table 11.1	Risk factor stratification
Low (apparently healthy)	Younger individuals (men under 45 and women under 55) who are asymptomatic and have no more than one risk factor
Moderate	Older individuals (men 45 or older and women 55 or older) or those with two or more risk factors
High	Individuals with one or more sign/symptom of Coronary Heart Disease (CHD) or those with known cardiovascular, pulmonary or metabolic disease

Larger health and fitness organisations should, by law, make a health and safety policy statement available to all staff and provide employees with relevant training. However, prior to working in any health and fitness environment the instructor must be familiar with several fundamental safety issues. It is in the interest of the instructor to identify and familiarise themselves with the Normal Operating Procedures (NOPs) (this often includes such things as security procedures and day to day operations) and Emergency Operating Procedures (EOPs) (such as fire and medical emergency) in the workplace to become aware of procedures that could help to minimise the occurrence of accident or injury. If an instructor is unsure of any health and safety concern, they should always contact their immediate line supervisor in order to clarify the issue. This is also the case should an instructor feel that procedures do not reflect health and safety regulations in some way.

Equipment management

The management of equipment during an exercise session is important with respect to overall safety. Equipment should not form an obstruction to the participants who are in the facility. For example, free weights should always be returned to their correct storage rack. It is also important to check equipment, such as pulleys and cables, for any wear and tear or malfunction prior to use. Instructors should also know how to operate any equipment and be able to locate manufacturers' manuals or guides. These guides should indicate the type and frequency of maintenance required. The facilities guidelines for the use of equipment are usually found in the NOPs along with relevant paperwork such as Gym Maintenance Report Sheets and faulty equipment notices.

Risk assessment

All health and fitness facilities have hazards and risks therefore it is the purpose of risk assessment to identify any that might be present. Hazards can come in the form of equipment left lying around or substances that are used for cleaning, etc., that are not stored or used correctly. In this case there is guidance in the form of Control of Substances Hazardous to Health Regulations which all facilities should have. Certain exercises can also constitute a risk depending on the individual concerned in terms of injury or disability. Although risks cannot be eradicated completely, they can be recognised, addressed and minimised. When planning an exercise session, it is advisable to complete and document a risk assessment. This acts as a written reminder for the instructor as well as providing evidence that preventative steps were taken, should an accident occur. Fig. 11.3 provides a template that can be used to formulate and document a basic risk assessment.

Emergency situations

As mentioned previously, instructors should be familiar with the facilities EOPs and how to report them. If problems occur during any emergency (such as a fire exit was locked), this should also be reported by the instructor to the appointed facility health and safety officer. If an emergency occurs during an exercise session, the instructor should follow the procedure below:

1. **Assess the situation.** Approach quickly but remain calm as casualties are often in distress. Identify any risks to yourself, the casualties and bystanders.
2. **Make the area safe.** The conditions that caused the emergency may need to be made safe.
3. **Give emergency aid.** Assess the casualty and give first aid.

Fig. 11.3	Example Risk Assessment Form		
Potential risk	Method of minimising risk	Action to be taken	Done
Recovery from shoulder injury	Limit range of motion and weight	Set pec dec range to start at limited range of motion	✓
Trips due to free-weights on floor in gym area	Ensure members return free-weights to storage when finished	Signs put up around gym area to instruct members to return free-weights.	✓
Slippage on floor space around water fountain.	Wipe floor regularly with paper towel.	Add this to daily cleaning rota.	✓

4. **Get help.** Send someone for help or telephone for assistance.
5. **Comfort the casualty.** Comfort and reassure the casualty until help arrives.

When contacting the emergency services, clear and accurate information must be given with regards the following:

• Own name
• Nature of emergency
• Details of any casualty
• Time of emergency
• Facility details
• Contact number

First aid

Prior to the arrival of the emergency services, the instructor must deal with the emergency in the correct manner. Any requirement for emergency first aid must be given and any minor injuries (such as cuts, sprains, strains) can be dealt with accordingly, otherwise, the casualty must be made as comfortable as possible. All staff at the centre must be informed

about the arrival of the emergency services so that clear access can be prepared in advance. As a simple guideline, the following procedure should be adhered to during an emergency situation:

1. Inform the people involved about the correct emergency procedures.
2. Follow procedures in a calm but correct manner.
3. Maintain the safety of those involved at all times.
4. Clearly and accurately report any problems to a responsible colleague.
5. Make a detailed report of the incident afterwards.

According to the Health and Safety (First Aid) Regulations 1981, employers must provide adequate equipment and facilities to enable first aid to be carried out on sick or injured employees. This does not by law extend to customers using the facility, although instructors trained in first aid should make every attempt to administer first aid should the situation arise. A current first-aid certificate is required before acceptance onto the Register of Exercise Professionals. Also, facilities should have a visible notice of the details of any first aider on-site.

Accident/incident report

In the event of an accident or incident during a gym session in which the instructor is in charge, an accident/incident report must be completed as a record of the event. The facility at which the instructor is working must provide the relevant form. It is important that this form is completed at the earliest available opportunity so that an accurate recall of the event can be made.

Child protection

According to Her Majesty's Government, any adult who works with children has a responsibility to keep children safe and protect them from sexual, physical and emotional harm. Failure to do this could be regarded as neglect and could lead to prosecution. For full details regarding duty of care go to www. everychildmatters.gov.uk. Children can often become infatuated with instructor figures, which can sometimes be misconstrued as affection and lead to potential grooming and sexual abuse. Instructors should be aware of this and try to give equal attention to all children in a group situation and follow the golden rule of never being alone with children. Situations sometimes arise when a child approaches an instructor and divulges sensitive information about potential abuse by another adult. Even though this puts the instructor in a very delicate situation, it is not their responsibility to decide if child abuse or inappropriate behaviour has taken place. Therefore the incident must be reported immediately but confidentially, as not all accusations turn out to be true. All facilities should have relevant reporting procedures as not all instructors will feel confident in this area, therefore, they should be aware of who they should discuss concerns with and the limit of their own involvement.

EXAMPLE QUESTIONS

11.1 The PAR-Q is a screening questionnaire used to identify conditions prior to encouraging exercise at...
a) a vigorous level
b) a high intensity
c) a light to moderate intensity
d) all levels

11.2 The PAR-Q is a screening questionnaire which is valid for what period of time?
a) no time limit
b) 6 weeks
c) 6 months
d) 12 months

11.3 True or false? The PAR-Q is a confidential document.

True ☐   False ☐

11.4 Which of the following is classed as a risk factor in relation to 'family history'?
a) Myocardial Infarction (MI) or sudden death before age 45 in father, brother or son. Before age 65 in mother, sister or daughter.
b) Myocardial Infarction (MI) or sudden death before age 55 in father, brother or son. Before age 65 in mother, sister or daughter.
c) Myocardial Infarction (MI) or sudden death before age 55 in father, brother or son. Before age 75 in mother, sister or daughter.
d) Myocardial Infarction (MI) or sudden death before age 55 in father, brother or son. Before age 60 in mother, sister or daughter.

11.5 Which of the following is classed as a risk factor in relation to 'fypertension'?
a) Systolic pressure of 120mmhg or above, or diastolic of 80mmhg or above.
b) Systolic pressure of 140mmhg or above, or diastolic of 80mmhg or above.
c) Systolic pressure of 120mmhg or above, or diastolic of 90mmhg or above.
d) Systolic pressure of 140mmhg or above, or diastolic of 90mmhg or above.

EXAMPLE QUESTIONS cont.

11.6 Which of the following is classed as a risk factor in relation to 'obesity'?
a) Body Mass Index of 15kg/m^2 or above.
b) Body Mass Index of 20kg/m^2 or above.
c) Body Mass Index of 25kg/m^2 or above.
d) Body Mass Index of 30kg/m^2 or above.

11.7 Which of the following is classed as a risk factor in relation to 'dyslipidemia'?
a) Total serum cholesterol of more than 3.2mmol/L
b) Total serum cholesterol of more than 6.2mmol/L
c) Total serum cholesterol of more than 5.2mmol/L
d) Total serum cholesterol of more than 4.2mmol/L

11.8 Which of the following is classed as a risk factor in relation to 'dyslipidemia'?
a) LDL more than 3.4mmol/L, or HDL less than 1.03mmol/L
b) LDL more than 3.2mmol/L, or HDL less than 1.03mmol/L
c) LDL more than 3.4mmol/L, or HDL less than 1.23mmol/L
d) LDL more than 4.4mmol/L, or HDL less than 1.03mmol/L

11.9 With regards to risk stratification, the ACSM state that people who are at moderate risk are...
a) Men 45 years or older and women 55 years or older or those with three or more risk factors.
b) Men 45 years or older and women 65 years or older or those with two or more risk factors.
c) Men 45 years or older and women 55 years or older or those with two or more risk factors.
d) Men 50 years or older and women 60 years or older or those with two or more risk factors.

EXAMPLE QUESTIONS cont.

11.10 Which of the following is classed as a risk factor in relation to 'impaired fasting glucose'?

a) 140mg/dL or more.

b) 80mg/dL or more.

c) 100mg/dL or more

d) 120mg/dL or more

11.11 The Health and Safety at Work Act (HSWA) 1974 outlines which of the following as roles of the instructor?

a) take responsible care for their own safety and that of others.

b) co-operate with employers in matters of safety.

c) both A and B

d) neither A nor B

11.12 True or false? The Health and Safety (First Aid) Regulations 1981 states that employers provide adequate equipment and facilities to enable first aid to be carried out on employees but not necessarily customers using the facility.

True ☐   False ☐

Further reading

American College of Sports Medicine (2009) *ACSM Guidelines to Exercise Testing and Prescription* (8th ed.), Lippincott, Williams & Wilkins

Baechle, R.T. (2008) *Essentials of Strength Training and Conditioning* (3rd ed.), Human Kinetics

HM Government (2004) *Children Act 2004*, HMSO

HM Government (2003) *Every Child Matters*, HMSO

HM Government (2006) *Working Together to Safeguard Children: A guide to inter-agency working to safeguard and promote the welfare of children*, HMSO

Howley, E.T. and Franks, B.D. (2003) *Health Fitness Instructor's Handbook* (4th ed.) Human Kinetics

Sewell, D., Watkins, P. and Griffin, M. (2005) *Sport and Exercise Science: An Introduction*, Hodder Arnold

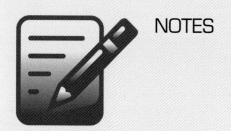

NOTES

BEHAVIOURAL CHANGE AND GOAL SETTING

OBJECTIVES

After completing this chapter, you will be able to:

1 Briefly discuss psychology in relation to exercise.

2 List and describe the stages of the Prochaska and DiClemente 'Stages of Change Model'.

3 List and describe the cognitive and behavioural processes relating to the stages of change model.

4 Relate the cognitive and behavioural processes to the appropriate stage of change.

5 List various motivational factors relating to individuals initiating or maintaining an exercise programme.

6 Explain how goal setting can be used in an exercise environment.

7 Describe the 'balance of good health plate model' in relation to healthy eating and relating to government key messages.

8 Describe the functions of certain nutrients including fluid, minerals and vitamins.

9 Briefly describe what is meant by the energy equation.

Level 2: Instructing Exercise and Fitness Knowledge

Basic Anatomy and Physiology

■ The importance of careful and thorough planning and preparation for sessions.

■ How to identify and agree objectives for the session based upon collected information.

■ The goals of the designated programmes that you are helping to deliver.

■ The needs and potential of the participants, including reasons for and barriers to participation in the appropriate activity.

Level 3: Instructing Physical Activity and Exercise Knowledge

Behaviour Change

■ Individual history and attitude to exercise:
  - Identifying and understanding the psychological benefits of exercise
  - Identifying the potential barriers to exercise participation

- • Principles of behaviour change: the 'Stages of Change Model' (Prochaska and DiClemente)
- • Determinants of behaviour change and the cognitive and behavioural processes to progress through the stages of change
- • Motivational and exercise adherence strategies:
  - • programming/prescription strategies
  - • the principles of motivational interviewing
  - • behavioral and outcome goal setting
  - • social support
  - • social reinforcement
  - • attentional strategies.

- ■ Intervention/motivational methods appropriate for each stage of behaviour change:
  - • Understanding why people relapse and relapse prevention strategies

Introduction

This chapter deals with the common processes of behavioural change and also goal-setting strategies in relation to guidelines within the National Occupational Standards framework for health and fitness. Within this framework, Level 2 and 3 instructors should be able to identify and describe common processes of behavioural change, as well as describe general methods of goal setting within the health and fitness industry.

Later chapters in the book provide information about programme design that, along with the content covered in this chapter, provides the instructor with the understanding and ability to design appropriate exercise programmes for apparently healthy individuals, in line with current guidelines for exercise.

Exercise psychology

As well as the physiological benefits of exercise, there are many psychological benefits that play an important part in helping individuals to take up and maintain a regular programme of exercise. The psychological effects of exercise can be difficult to measure; however, it is claimed anecdotally that exercise can improve subjective feelings such as self-esteem, mood, self-image and confidence. It is also thought that exercise can help to reduce stress and anxiety by providing a distraction.

Even though there are possible physiological explanations for these psychological effects, such as endorphins released after exercise having a positive effect on mood, psychological strategies about exercise are considered to play an important role in uptake and adherence to exercise. One of the main areas of focus from a psychological perspective is finding strategies to help individuals overcome barriers to exercise by making permanent changes to their lifestyle and behaviour. These barriers include lack of funds, poor self-image, lack of enjoyment and, primarily, lack of available time. Instructors within the health and fitness industry might choose to identify which barriers to exercise are relevant to their particular client by simply asking direct questions. Once these barriers have been identified, the instructor can devise strategies to help overcome them. For example, if lack of time is an issue, the instructor could suggest walking more briskly whenever there is a need to walk, or getting off the bus one stop earlier if the client uses public transport. The instructor could also choose to use psychological strategies that have been successful following many years of research. One such strategy is the 'Behavioural Change Model' discussed below.

Behaviour change

Much of the adult population does not engage in any form of regular exercise; therefore, starting an exercise programme often requires a change in lifestyle and habits on the part of the individual. This is sometimes known as *behavioural change*. It can be challenging for both the individual and the instructor to overcome habits that have been in place for many years, as research has suggested that behavioural change is a long-term process. However, models such as Prochaska and DiClemente's *Stages of Change Model* can help instructors to facilitate the process.

'Stages of Change Model'

This model proposes that there are a number of stages to any lifestyle change, such as stopping smoking or alcohol rehabilitation. Indeed, the research carried out by Prochaska and DiClemente used smoking cessation as the theme for the conception of the model; however, it can also be applied to exercise uptake.

As can be seen from Fig. 12.1, there are several stages of change that will vary in duration depending on the individual. Table 12.1 describes the stages of change in more detail.

It is interesting to note that stages of change in relation to exercise uptake are cyclical in nature: in other words, an individual can go from one stage to the next and back again without ever moving any further on in the model. Approximately 15 per cent of all individuals will experience relapse to the contemplation or pre-contemplation stage. Depending on which stage of the model the individual is at, it can be

Fig. 12.1 The 'Stages of Change Model'

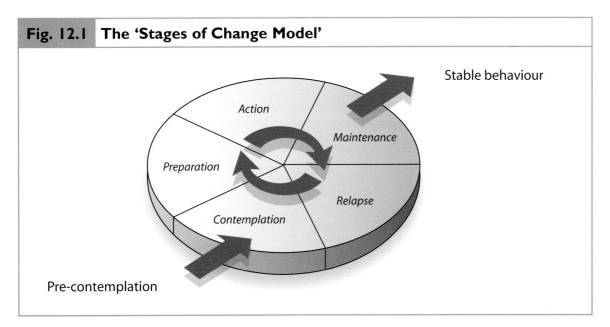

Stable behaviour

Action

Maintenance

Preparation

Relapse

Contemplation

Pre-contemplation

Table 12.1	Description of the 'Stages of Change' (Prochaska and DiClemente)
Stage	Description
Pre-contemplation (I won't)	The individual does not intend to take any action in the short term (within about six months)
Contemplation (I might)	The individual intends to take action soon but is unsure about the change
Preparation (I will)	The individual has taken steps towards action and is planning to act, usually within one month
Action (I am)	The individual has taken action and changed his/her behaviour in the short term
Maintenance (I have)	Behavioural change has lasted more than six months and the individual is committed to the change
Relapse	This can happen at any stage and many times over

important to provide help or support in order for the individual to progress through the stages. One of the strategies used for this purpose is that of *cognitive* and *behavioural processes.*

Cognitive and behavioural processes

The stage an individual is at can be ascertained by simple questioning during the screening and lifestyle sessions (see Chapter 11). Simply asking the individual which stage they think they are at is sometimes enough, or the answers they give to the instructor's questions can make it evident. Depending on the identified stage of change, the instructor can use strategies known as *cognitive* (experiential) and *behavioural processes* to help the individual, hopefully to arrive at the maintenance stage.

Cognitive processes involve implementing changes to the way individuals think about lifestyle and are divided into five areas (see Table 12.2).

NEED TO KNOW

The Stages of Change Model is also known as the *trans-theoretical model.*

The cognitive processes outlined in Table 12.2 are usually adopted by individuals in the early stages of the Stages of Change Model, (pre-contemplation to preparation). Once the individual has moved to the action or maintenance stage, the cognitive processes are not as important, as the individual has already thought about the exercise. At this stage the five *behavioural processes* listed in Table 12.3 can be more important.

Depending on which stage the individual is at, certain cognitive or behavioural processes are more likely to be successful in helping

Table 12.2	Cognitive processes
Cognitive processes	Description
Consciousness-raising (increasing knowledge)	This relates to seeking new information and understanding, such as ascertaining the benefits of exercise and the risks associated with sedentary behaviour. In terms of health and fitness, examples include visiting one's GP or talking to friends.
Dramatic relief (warning signs)	This relates to the feelings that can be experienced as a result of exercise or sedentary behaviour, such as injury or pain, or tasks becoming more difficult as the individual ages.
Environmental re-evaluation	This involves reflecting on how behaviour can affect other people, such as being a role model and helping others, or sedentary behaviour 'rubbing off' on a friend or partner.
Self re-evaluation	This can be related to re-educating the individual about beliefs related to exercise, such as exercise does not need to be painful to have good benefits, or it can prevent another heart attack.
Social liberation	This relates to helping oneself or others in similar situations and increasing awareness of exercise strategies.

them to move towards the next stage of change. Table 12.4 will guide the instructor to employ the most useful processes at various stages of change.

NEED TO KNOW

Many professional sports clubs employ psychologists to help implement motivational strategies.

Even though research is limited in the health and fitness environment in relation to exercise uptake, there is much anecdotal evidence to support the use of the processes. However, instructors should be aware of and focus on the move from the contemplation stage to the action stage, as this is often reported to be the most difficult transition. Instructors should also be aware that many individuals will cite barriers that prevent them from exercising, such as lack of funds, lack of transport, no peer support and self-consciousness, among others. Therefore, it is the role of the instructor to devise strategies and suggest ways for the individual to overcome these potential barriers.

The psychological strategies discussed in this chapter have been shown to influence exercise adherence and, as such, positively impact on the benefits of a healthy lifestyle. As these psychological strategies extend beyond the scope of this book, instructors and individuals are encouraged to increase their knowledge of

Table 12.3	Behavioural processes
Behavioural processes	**Description**
Self-liberation (understanding the benefits)	This relates to experiencing the benefits of committing to exercise by taking responsibility, which can inspire confidence and self-belief. At this stage the instructor and the individual should make firm resolutions.
Helping relationships	This relates to providing and accepting support for the individual and encouraging empowerment. Buddy systems or personal trainers can be used here. Remind the individual why exercise can be good.
Reinforcement management (rewards)	This involves providing rewards such as T-shirts, badges and certificates for meeting goals and targets, and punishment or forfeits for not.
Counter-conditioning (alternatives)	This involves trying to focus on the positive changes of exercise choices replacing sedentary choices, such as using stairs instead of lifts or walking the dog instead of watching TV.
Stimulus control	This involves trying to remove options for sedentary behaviour, such as hiding the TV remote control, switching on the radio as opposed to the TV and keeping exercise clothes prominent.

this particular area as part of self-development and progression. There are many sources available to the instructor (or individual) such as books, websites and courses that relate specifically to the health and fitness industry, in particular to areas such as exercise adherence, performance enhancement, teambuilding, lifestyle management and injury rehabilitation.

TASK

List the stages of change and explain how various cognitive and behavioural strategies can help individuals to move through the stages.

Motivation

The word 'motivate' is derived from the Latin for 'move' and can be defined as 'the internal mechanisms and external stimuli that arouse and direct our behaviour'. In other words, motivation is what prompts a person to act. This can include the motivation to make lifestyle changes in order to affect weight loss or increase cardiovascular fitness, which relates directly to the cognitive and behavioural processes discussed previously.

In relation to exercise, individuals might have more than one motive to start or maintain an exercise programme, and their motivation could change over a period of time. Many

Table 12.4	Processes most likely to aid movement towards the next 'stage of change'		
Contemplation	Preparation	Action	Maintenance
Consciousness raising: statistics on obesity, information about how exercise can reduce obesity, etc.	Self re-evaluation: small lifestyle changes can have benefits, etc.	Self-liberation: congratulations, you did it and it feels good!	Reinforcement management: well done, you've won a T-shirt for achieving your first goal
Dramatic relief: sedentary behaviour makes you feel lethargic but exercise makes you feel good, etc.			Helping relationships: train with a partner – this really helps
Environmental re-evaluation: friends might want to join you, etc.			Counter-conditioning: we have an agreement at work not to use the stairs, etc.
			Stimulus control: my partner only allows the remote after exercise, etc.

factors can affect motivational preference, so instructors must be aware that they need to regularly address this with the individual. Table 12.5 outlines some of the commonly cited motives for individuals who are either just starting an exercise programme or maintaining an exercise programme.

Types of motivation

Various motivational factors can influence training in different ways. Athletes may be highly motivated for competition reasons, whereas a beginner may be motivated by factors such as weight loss. These motivational

Table 12.5	Common motives for starting/maintaining an exercise programme	
Starting		Maintaining
Health		Enjoyment
Appearance		Role model's influence
Guidance		Variation of activities
Challenge		Social
Submission		Self-esteem
Compulsion		Helping others
Fitness		

factors may come from external sources such as a coach or a partner, or from internal factors such as the individual themselves. These types of motivation are commonly referred to as *extrinsic* and *intrinsic* motivation.

Extrinsic motivation

This term is used when individuals are motivated to exercise by external rewards such as certificates, T-shirts, medals and trophies. Many people are motivated extrinsically, so it is prudent to ascertain which extrinsic motivational factors an individual responds best to. However, external rewards can be motivational providing they are not the only reason for taking part in exercise. For adherence reasons, it is also important to make sure that individuals are not over-reliant on external rewards but focus on internal motivational factors as well.

Intrinsic motivation

This term is used when individuals are motivated to exercise by factors such as enjoyment, fun or self-satisfaction. This type of motivation can be linked to outcome goals (see page 199): for example, when an individual achieves a certain exercise goal it could lead to a positive feeling of self-achievement. It might be beneficial to try and identify the type of motivational strategy that might suit the individual during the initial consultation. This can be done by questioning the individual about past exercise history and the success or failure of that exercise history. If a motivational preference cannot be established, try employing motivational techniques, such as those listed below, to assess if they have a positive or negative effect.

Common motivational techniques

Below are some common motivational techniques to try with clients.

1. To start with, set short-term goals that are easily achievable.
2. Encourage the individual to find a training partner (use a buddy system).
3. Keep an exercise diary for visual effect.
4. If weight loss is a goal, use pictures of the individual when he or she was slimmer as an incentive to get back to that size.
5. Keep a reminder in a prominent place (on the individual's desk or fridge door) of the reasons why the individual wants to achieve their specific goals: for example, wanting to increase cardio fitness to run in a charity fun run in six months time.
6. Introduce the individual to other activities and social events within the exercise facility.
7. Encourage the individual to keep their exercise kit in a prominent place.

TASK

Briefly define the term 'motivation' and list the various extrinsic and intrinsic motivational techniques that are commonly used in the health and fitness industry.

Goal setting

Goal setting is a simple, yet often misused motivational technique that can provide some structure for an exercise programme. Goals are usually set in order to accomplish a specific task in a specific period of time, such as losing a certain amount of weight for a wedding or being able to run a half marathon in six months

Table 12.6	Common process and outcome goals
Process goals	**Outcome goals**
• Be able to do free-weight exercises • Be able to run or jog without heart pounding • Establish a routine • Enjoy the exercise • Exercise on your own	• Reduce body fat percentage • Decrease blood pressure • Increase VO$_2$ max • Complete a marathon • Reduce a dress size

time. Goal setting can provide a plan of action to help the individual to focus and direct their activities. Information gathered during screening can help the instructor and client to set specific goals that are individualised and relevant to that client. Generally speaking, in relation to exercise there are two categories of goal setting: process goals and outcome goals. Process goals are goals where the skill is broken down into manageable units for the subject to focus on. Often, form and technique can be classed as process goals as they are task-related rather than results-related. Outcome goals are concerned only with the ultimate outcome, for example, success or failure, winning or losing. In other words, outcome goals are results-related as opposed to task-related. Focus on outcome goals can often affect attention to process goals, which can result in a detrimental effect on the outcome. Therefore, instructors and individuals should try to focus on process goals as well as outcome goals in the initial stages of an exercise programme. Typical process and outcome goals are outlined in Table 12.6.

The SMARTER principle

Goals in relation to exercise can be set for the short, medium and long term. If only long-term goals were set, the individual might lose interest and exercise adherence could be affected, while achievement of short-term goals could act as a motivational tool for the individual. When agreeing goals with the individual, whether short-, medium- or long-term, the acronym *SMART* or *SMARTER* is a useful guide and includes several common characteristics that are often associated with effective goal setting (see Table 12.7).

Regardless of the goals that are set, the instructor and client must review these goals on a regular basis in order to make any changes that are necessary. It is often the case that changes must be made in relation to the lifestyle commitments of the client but changes should also be made if the instructor feels that the client is not 'on-track' to achieve the set goals. Fitness testing is a common method of judging where the client is in terms of their programme. For information on health and fitness testing refer to *Practical Fitness Testing* by Morc Coulson and Dave Archer.

Healthy eating

In terms of goal setting, as well as focusing on activity prescription, many instructors like to give advice or set specific goals relating to nutrition or dietary habits but it should be stressed that the amount of information should be limited to key areas which follow current government guidelines. For information or

Table 12.7	Examples of SMARTER goals	
S	Goals must be **Specific**	If an individual wants to follow a weight-loss programme, be specific about the amount of weight loss that is set as the target. For instance, 0.5 kg per week could be a specific target.
M	Training targets should be **Measurable**	In the example above, 0.5 kg per week is a measurable amount, as opposed to 'lose a little weight each week'.
A	Goals should be **Adjustable**	If an individual finds the target too easy or too hard, the instructor must adapt the programme to suit. In other words, the programme must be adjustable.
R	Goals must be **Realistic**	Set targets that are achievable: 0.5 kg weight loss per week is an achievable target for most people, whereas a target of over 3 kg per week might not be achievable by all people.
T	Training targets should be **Time-based**	For example, 0.5 kg weight loss per week can be a short-term target that can lead to an overall loss of about 26 kg a year, which is a long-term goal.
E	Goals should be challenging and **Exciting**	The chances of adherence to the programme are much greater if the programme is exciting in some way.
R	Goals should be **Recorded**	Make sure that the individual keeps a record of exercise activity as this provides a visual stimulus for the individual and prevents any confusion over a longer term.

advice beyond these key messages, instructors should refer clients to qualified people such as state registered dieticians. One of the main sources of information relating to healthy eating is that of the government *Balance of Good Health* otherwise known as the 'Plate Model' as shown in Fig 12.2. Dietary goals should always be limited to the advice contained within this model.

The Plate Model

The government has produced this simple visual way of educating the public about a healthy diet.

The plate model concentrates on five commonly accepted food groups (rather than individual nutrients) and the proportions of these foods that should be eaten from each group:

- Bread, other cereals and potatoes: for example, bread, cereals, potatoes, rice, noodles, pasta.
- Fruit and vegetables: for example, apple, banana, grapes, kiwi, cabbage, peppers, sweet corn, peas.
- Milk and dairy foods: for example, milk, cheese and yoghurt.

- Meat, fish and alternatives: for example, chicken, beef, cod, prawns, eggs, chick peas, nuts
- Foods containing fat and foods containing sugar: for example, biscuits, jam, margarine, mayonnaise, confectionery, crisps

The intended message is that people should choose a variety of foods from the four largest groups every day. More foods should be eaten from the bread, other cereals and potatoes group and the fruit and vegetables group compared with the milk and dairy foods group and the meat, fish and alternatives group. Foods in the smallest group (foods containing fat and containing sugar) should be used sparingly if they are eaten every day or not eaten too often.

Fluid

Water is considered to be the most important nutrient as it makes up between 40 and 70 per cent of total body mass (depending on age, gender and body composition). Many metabolic processes in the body require water to be present, especially digestion and absorption of nutrients and this can be affected if the body becomes too dehydrated. As water is lost through processes such as urination, exhalation and evaporation through the skin, etc., it must be replaced on a daily basis in the form of food (many foods contain water, especially fruits) and fluids. The Plate Model does show some fluids, such as milk and fruit juice, however, water, tea and coffee are major contributors to fluid intake (not alcohol). Even though there is no exact recommendation about the amount

Fig. 12.2 The Balance of Good Health Plate Model

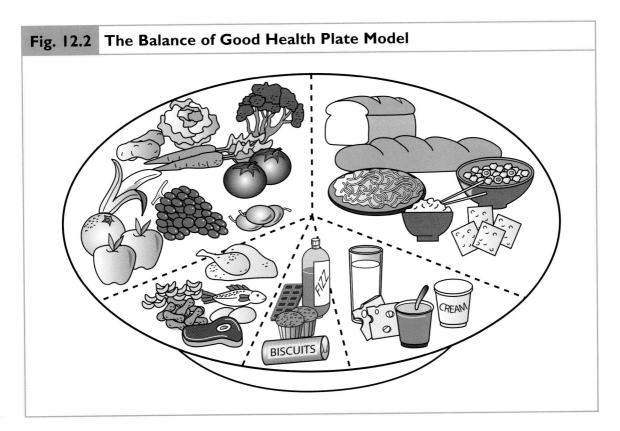

of total fluid that should be drunk in a day, a general guideline is 6–8 glasses, cups or mugs of fluid.

Preventing Dehydration

The body loses more water exercising than when at rest, but following simple guidelines can help to prevent dehydration.

- Do not rely on thirst to let you know when you need to drink, it is an unreliable indicator.
- Avoid overdressing as this can cause greater fluid losses, use breathable exercise clothing.
- Cut down on your intake of tea/coffee/ alcohol, these are all diuretics and cause the body to lose water.
- Check the colour of your urine on a regular basis, as this should be pale. A dark yellow/ orange indicates possible dehydration.

Nutrients

All foods contain chemicals known as nutrients which are needed for essential processes such as growth and metabolism. Nutrients needed in very small amounts are called micronutrients (vitamins, minerals and fibre) and those that are needed in larger quantities are called macronutrients (proteins, fats and carbohydrates). There are many guidelines in relation to the recommended amounts of macronutrients such as that by The World Health Organization, which suggests an average daily intake (based on the ideal amount of calories) of carbohydrate, fat and protein for the general population should be made up of the following:

- **Fats:** up to 30 per cent (less than 10 per cent from saturated fats)
- **Protein:** 10–15 per cent
- **Carbohydrates:** 55–60 per cent (less than 10 per cent from simple sugars)

All calories should come from macronutrients which should be balanced (as in the Plate Model) enough in the diet to provide the necessary amounts of micronutrients as well. Vitamins (listed in Table 12.8) are organic substances that are essential in the metabolism of fats, carbohydrates and protein and numerous other functions such as blood clotting, protein synthesis and bone formation.

Vitamins

Vitamins are normally categorised into two groups: fat-soluble (transported and stored with lipids) and water-soluble (not stored, transported in water). In most cases, the lack of a vitamin causes severe problems as shown in Table 12.8.

Minerals

There are a number of minerals (inorganic elements) that our bodies must have in order to create specific molecules needed in the body. Table 12.9 lists and describes the common functions of certain minerals. Minerals are often lacking in the diet which leads to various problems such as osteoporosis through lack of calcium intake and anaemia through lack of iron intake. Other minerals such as sodium are over consumed by many of the population. A high sodium intake has been linked to hypertension.

Energy balance

One of the main concerns resulting from lack of activity is that of overweight and obesity. This can be explained simply by using something known as the 'energy balance equation'. This is used to describe the balance

Table 12.8	Vitamin uses and effects of deficiency	
Vitamin	Main use	Deficiency
Vitamin A (fat soluble)	Retinol – found in plants such as carrots. Essential for vision in dim light and is also required for skin, mucous membranes and growth.	Night blindness (xerophthalmia)
Vitamin B (water soluble)	B1: Thiamine – release of energy from carbohydrates, especially important for the brain and nerve function. B2: Riboflavin – release of energy, especially from protein and fat B3: Niacin – energy release from nutrients B5: Pantothenic acid – utilised in metabolic pathways. B6: Pyridoxine – used in many biological reactions is especially associated with amino acid metabolism. B7: Biotin – cell growth and fat metabolism. B9: Folic Acid–important for protecting the new foetus. B12: Cyanocobalamin – important for folate metabolism.	Beriberi (nervous system disorder). Problems with lips, tongue, skin. Pellagra (skin disorder). Fatigue. Skin problems. Hair loss, dermatitis. Diarrhoea, anaemia. Pernicious anaemia.
Vitamin C (water soluble)	Ascorbic acid – immune system, aids wound healing and iron absorption.	Scurvy (sickness and skin disorders)
Vitamin D (fat soluble)	Calciferol – Promotes calcium absorption from food.	Rickets (bone softening)
Vitamin E (fat soluble)	Tocopherol – protective effect for cell membranes.	Malabsorption of fats, anaemia.
Vitamin K (fat soluble)	Menaquinone – especially required to produce blood clotting proteins.	Poor blood clotting, internal bleeding.

between energy intake (in the form of food) and energy expenditure (in terms of energy stores used for normal function and activity) on a daily basis. Fig. 12.3 shows that if the amount of energy taken in is greater than the amount of energy expended then it is likely that the excess energy will result in weight gain. Conversely if the amount of energy taken in is less than the amount of energy expended then this could result in weight loss.

Table 12.9	Common functions of minerals
Mineral	Common function
Calcium	Used by teeth, bones. Muscle and nerve activity. Blood clotting.
Chloride	Metabolism (the process of turning food into energy).
Copper	Oxygen transportation.
Fluorine	Strengthens teeth.
Iron	Transports oxygen in red blood cells. Protein metabolism.
Iodine	Thyroid function, metabolism, growth and energy production.
Magnesium	Used in enzyme activity and muscle function. Protein building.
Manganese	Has a role in the body's anti-oxidant defences.
Molybdenum	Involved in the metabolism of DNA.
Phosphorus	Present in bones and teeth, a component of all cells.
Potassium	Important for brain and nerve function.
Selenium	Anti-oxidant, growth and metabolism, pancreas function.
Sodium	Regulation of body water content and nerve function.
Zinc	Growth and repair, taste perception, anti-oxidant, foetal development.

Fig. 12.3 The energy balance equation

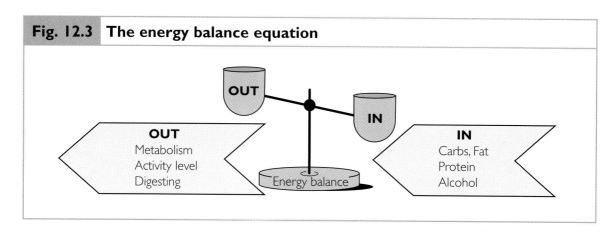

EXAMPLE QUESTIONS

12.1 The 'stages of change' model follows what type of pattern?
a) rhythmical
b) cyclical
c) exponential
d) linear

12.2 Approximately what percentage of all individuals will experience relapse back to the contemplation or pre-contemplation stage?
a) 5%
b) 10%
c) 15%
d) 20%

12.3 True or false? Cognitive processes are usually adopted by individuals in the early stages of the 'stages of change model' from not thinking about exercise to the action of taking up exercise.

True ☐   False ☐

12.4 True or false? Behavioural processes are usually adopted by individuals in the later stages of the 'stages of change model'.

True ☐   False ☐

12.5 What is the following a definition of? *'The internal mechanisms and external stimuli which arouse and direct our behaviour'.*
a) cognitive process
b) behavioural process
c) goal setting
d) motivation

EXAMPLE QUESTIONS cont.

12.6 Which term is used to describe when an individual is motivated to exercise by factors such as enjoyment, fun or self-satisfaction?
a) intrinsic motivation
b) extrinsic motivation
c) external motivation
d) behavioural motivation

12.7 When a skill is broken down into manageable units that the subject can focus on, it is otherwise known as what type of goal?
a) SMART
b) outcome
c) process
d) realistic

12.8 The World Health Organization suggests an average daily intake of carbohydrate, fat and protein for the general population should be made up of which of the following?
a) 30% fat, 5–10% protein, 50–55% carbohydrates
b) 30% fat, 10–15% protein, 55–60% carbohydrates
c) 20% fat, 10–15% protein, 60–65% carbohydrates
d) 10% fat, 15–20% protein, 55–60% carbohydrates

12.9 Which of the following vitamins is considered to be important for promoting calcium absorption from food?
a) A
b) K
c) D
d) C

12.10 Which of the following vitamins is considered to be important for producing blood clotting proteins?
a) A
b) K
c) D
d) C

EXAMPLE QUESTIONS cont.

12.11 Which of the following minerals is considered to be important for brain and nerve function?

a) sodium

b) potassium

c) selenium

d) zinc

12.12 Which of the following minerals is considered to be important for the regulation of body water content and nerve function?

a) sodium

b) potassium

c) selenium

d) zinc

Further reading

American College of Sports Medicine (2009) *ACSM Guidelines to Exercise Testing and Prescription* (8th ed.), Lippincott, Williams & Wilkins

Arthritis Research Campaign (2002) *Arthritis: The big picture*, Arthritis Research Campaign.

Atkinson, R. and Hilgard, E.R. (2003) *Introduction to Psychology* (14th ed.), Wadsworth Publishing

Boutcher, S.H. (2000) 'Cognitive performance, fitness and ageing', in Biddle, S.J.H., Fox, K.R. and Boutcher, S.H., *Physical Activity and Psychological Well-Being*, Routledge, 118–129

British Heart Foundation Health Promotion Research Group (2005) *Coronary Heart Disease Statistics*, Department of Public Health

Bull, S.J., (2000) *Sport Psychology: A self-help*, Crowood

Butler, R.J. (2000) *Sport Psychology in Performance*. NY: Oxford University Press.

Cox, R.H. (1998) *Sport Psychology Concepts and Applications*, Brown & Benchmark

Department of Health (2000) *Coronary Heart Disease: National Service Framework for coronary heart disease – modern standards and service models*, Department of Health

Department of Health (2004) *At Least 5 a Week: Evidence on the impact of physical activity and its relationship to health*, Department of Health

Department of Health, Health Survey for England (2007) *Healthy Lifestyles: Knowledge, attitudes and behaviour*, NHS Information Centre for Health and Social Care

Duda, J.L. (1998) *Advances in Sport and Exercise Psychology Measurement*, Fitness Information Technology Inc.

Howley, E.T. and Franks, B.D. (2003) *Health Fitness Instructor's Handbook* (4th ed.) Human Kinetics

Kugler, J., Seelbach, H. and Kruskemper, G.M. (1994) 'Effects of rehabilitation exercise programmes on anxiety and depression in coronary patients: a meta-analysis', *British Journal of Clinical Psychology*, 33: 401–410

McArdle, W.D., Katch, F.I. and Katch, V.L. (2007) *Exercise Physiology* (6th ed.), Lippincott, Williams & Wilkins

NHS Information Centre, Lifestyle Statistics (2009) *Statistics on Obesity, Physical Activity and Diet: England, February 2009*, NHS Information Centre for Health and Social Care

Orlick, T. (1998) *Embracing Your Potential*, Human Kinetics

Van Staa, T.P., Dennison, E.M., Leufkens, H.G. and Cooper, C. (2001) 'Epidemiology of fractures in England and Wales', *Bone*, 29: 517–522

Weinberg, R. and Gould, D (2000) *Foundations of Sport and Exercise Psychology*, Human Kinetics.

World Health Organization (2002) *The World Health Report 2002. Reducing risks, promoting healthy life*, WHO Press

NOTES

COMPONENTS AND INDUCTION OF AN EXERCISE SESSION

13

OBJECTIVES

After completing this chapter, you will be able to:

1 Explain the term 'induction' in relation to exercise sessions.

2 Describe the process of warm-up, cardio, cool-down, and resistance and flexibility inductions for beginners to exercise.

3 List the common guidelines relating to the use of cardiovascular equipment.

4 List and describe the components of an exercise session.

5 List and describe each of the 'cardio training zones'.

6 Briefly describe the terms 'interval' and 'fartlek' in relation to cardio training.

7 Describe the term 'resistance exercise continuum'.

8 Explain the term 'periodisation' and list its components.

Level 2: Instructing Exercise and Fitness Knowledge

Basic Anatomy and Physiology

- The application of the principles and variables of fitness to the components of fitness.

- How to apply the principles and variables of fitness to a range of activities that will achieve various health benefits and the required fitness development.

- The importance of careful and thorough planning and preparation for sessions.

- The goals of the designated programmes that you are helping to deliver.

- How to apply the principles and variables of fitness to a range of activities that will achieve various health benefits and the required fitness development.

- The programme/session card and how to record plans on it.

Level 3: Instructing Physical Activity and Exercise Knowledge

Components of fitness
- Heart-rate training zones

- Components of fitness:
  - Aerobic capacity
  - Muscular strength
  - Muscular resistance
  - Flexibility
- Rep ranges for strength, power, endurance and hypertrophy
- ACSM guidelines for developing each component of fitness
- Continuum between muscular strength and muscular endurance
- Interval and fartlek training – principles and practice
- Principles of periodisation
  - Macro-, meso- and micro-cycles
  - Volume vs intensity through the cycles
- Importance of rest and signs and symptoms of overtraining

Introduction

This chapter deals with the components of an exercise session in relation to guidelines within the National Occupational Standards framework for health and fitness. Level 2 and 3 instructors should be able to identify the components of an exercise session and list the guidelines associated with them.

This chapter, along with others in the book, provides information regarding the practical application of theoretical knowledge. This will allow the instructor to design appropriate exercise programmes for apparently healthy individuals, in line with current guidelines for exercise.

Components of an exercise session

A typical exercise session forming part of an overall exercise programme would normally include the following components,

as recommended by the American College of Sports Medicine:

1. Warm-up
2. Conditioning phase (including cardio, resistance and flexibility training)
3. Cool-down.

Warm-up

Prior to the exercise session, it is essential that the body (and in particular the connective tissues) is fully warmed in order to reduce the potential for injury. Research has shown that perhaps the main factor in muscular injury prevention is muscle temperature (Noonan, 1993): muscle is more elastic when warm and therefore less susceptible to injury.

The entire warm-up should take about 5–10 minutes and should facilitate the transition from rest to the level of exercise required in the main session. The intensity of the warm-up should increase gradually in order to avoid the onset of oxygen debt (see page 38) and can be performed using cardiovascular equipment, such as a treadmill, rower, cycle or step machine or, if no equipment is available, through brisk walking or slow jogging. There is very little difference in the benefits of each method, as they are all capable of stressing the cardiorespiratory system.

The warm-up should aim to achieve a change in a number of physiological responses, in order that the body can work safely and effectively. Typical benefits of a warm-up are:

1. An increase in body temperature, specifically core muscle temperature
2. An increase in the elasticity of muscular tissues
3. A decreased risk of soft-tissue injury
4. Activation of the neuromuscular system
5. An increase in mental alertness.

Conditioning phase

According to the ACSM, the conditioning phase of an exercise session should include one or more of the following types of training: cardiovascular, resistance and flexibility. For a comprehensive session, all areas are recommended.

Cardiovascular training

The cardiovascular session should follow on from the warm-up and can involve the same type of cardiovascular equipment. At the end of the warm-up the heart rate should be at the level required for the cardiovascular session, depending on the goal of the individual. Guidelines for the recommended heart-rate levels and duration and frequency of exercise can be taken from the ACSM guidelines (see Chapter 12).

Benefits of cardiovascular training

The main benefits of cardiovascular training, dependant on the intensity, frequency and duration of the exercise, are:

1. Weight (fat) loss due to an increase in fat metabolism
2. Increased glycogen stores
3. Increased aerobic and anaerobic enzymes
4. Increase in the number and size of mitochondria
5. Increased number of capillaries
6. Increased myoglobin levels
7. Increased recruitment of muscle fibres
8. Increased self-confidence and self-esteem.

NEED TO KNOW

For an average individual, it is recommended that energy expenditure per day from exercise should be between 300 and 400 kcal.

Cardio training zones

When prescribing cardiovascular exercise, the intensity (how hard the individual should exercise) should be carefully considered. Before agreeing the level of the exercise with an individual, it is useful to understand the benefits of exercising at different levels of intensity, otherwise known as *cardio training zones* (see Fig. 13.1). In basic terms, each specific training zone is related to a heart-rate range in which certain benefits might be expected. The zones are not exact, but they are useful as a guide to cardiovascular training as the benefits relating to each zone are reasonably accurate.

Training zones are based on a percentage window (60–70 per cent, for example) of

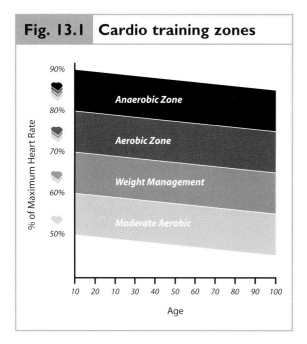

Fig. 13.1 Cardio training zones

maximum heart rate (MHR). Within each training zone, subtle physiological effects take place in relation to the heart rate.

Moderate aerobic zone: 50–60 per cent MHR

This training zone is mainly suitable for deconditioned individuals, or individuals who cannot maintain a normal conversation within the heart-rate levels specific to this zone. Regular exercise in this zone will lead to slight improvements in cardiovascular function, depending on the frequency and duration of the exercise undertaken.

Exercise sessions within this zone might only last for a few minutes, so the minimum goal of 20 minutes of cardiovascular exercise, as recommended by the ACSM, should become a target for the client to achieve comfortably before progressing to higher intensity levels such as those in the weight-management zone.

Weight-management zone: 60–70 per cent MHR

Training within this zone develops endurance and aerobic capacity, again depending on the frequency and duration of the exercise undertaken. Exercising in this zone also burns fat at a higher rate then the previous zone, which is associated with weight loss. There should also be an overall improvement in the health status and cardiorespiratory function of the individual.

At this level of intensity, most individuals will be aware of an increase in heart rate, but should be able to carry out a normal conversation. The weight-management zone should be achievable for most beginners to exercise and should be sufficient to bring about overload and hence adaptation to the demands of the exercise. From an exercise adherence perspective, this zone can be beneficial to beginners in that they should feel reasonably comfortable with the level of intensity but should also experience the benefits of adaptation. As the benefits of cardiovascular exercise are affected by frequency, duration and intensity, it is suggested that duration should follow the ACSM guidelines of 20–60 minutes, at a frequency of 3–5 days per week. In terms of intensity, a greater amount of energy will be expended at 70 per cent of maximum heart rate compared to that expended at 60 per cent for the same amount of time; this will affect the overall amount of fat used as fuel for the exercise.

Aerobic zone: 70–80 per cent MHR

This zone is sometimes referred to as the 'fitness' zone and can also be described as the moderate-to-vigorous intensity zone. The ability of the body to transport oxygen to and carbon dioxide away from the working muscles can be developed and improved by training in this zone. At this level of intensity breathing rate is increased, so this level is more appropriate for individuals who are used to exercising on a regular basis. Some individuals will still be able to carry out a conversation at this level, but others might find it difficult to do so while still maintaining regular breathing.

Anaerobic zone: 80–90 per cent MHR

Training in this zone can help to develop the lactic acid system (see Chapter 6). In this zone the individual's anaerobic threshold is normally reached. The amount of fat utilised (in percentage terms) as the main source of energy in this zone is greatly reduced, as glycogen stored in the muscle is the predominant source of fuel. One of the by-products of using glycogen as a fuel is lactic acid. The body can normally remove and deal with low levels of lactic acid, but as levels of lactic acid start to increase the body reaches a point at which it can no longer remove the lactic acid from the working muscles quickly enough. This happens at a heart rate, and hence intensity, that is specific to each individual and is usually accompanied by a rapid rise in heart rate and a slowing of intensity. This point is known as the *onset of blood lactate* or *OBLA*. The correct type of training can increase the body's ability to remove lactic acid for a longer period of time, thus delaying the OBLA. Due to the high-intensity levels associated with this zone, it is mainly suitable for athletes or those individuals who have a considerable base of fitness. It is important to note that at higher intensity levels such as these, the risk of orthopaedic injuries and cardiac complications is increased.

Duration of cardiovascular training

Regardless of the training zone being used, the guidelines for cardiovascular endurance as stated by the ACSM suggest a duration of 20–60 minutes continuous or intermittent exercise (intermittent meaning an accumulation of 10-minute bouts of exercise throughout the day). A distinction should be made between this definition and intermittent types of cardiovascular training that are sometimes used by individuals as a training method. Two common types of intermittent cardiovascular training are *fartlek* and *interval training*.

Fartlek

The term fartlek loosely translates as 'speed play' and involves alternating the intensity level throughout the duration of the cardiovascular session. This kind of training appears to be random in relation to recovery periods and intensity levels.

Interval training

Interval training is a more systematic form of training that uses precise work:recovery ratios. For example, an individual will maintain a constant speed for a certain period of time at an aerobic level, then increase the intensity to an anaerobic level for a short period of time. The intensity will then be reduced to a lower level than at the start to allow the individual to recover. The process then begins again.

There is a complex interaction between the exact levels of aerobic and anaerobic intensity and the period of recovery, and a number of sessions are normally required in order to fine-tune this. Fig. 13.2 provides an example of one cycle in an interval training session and can be explained as follows:

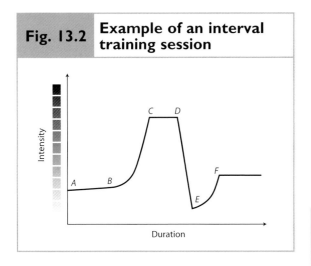

Fig. 13.2 Example of an interval training session

- **A–B:** This is the individual's normal level of aerobic intensity.
- **B–C:** The intensity is gradually increased to an anaerobic level.
- **C–D:** The anaerobic level is maintained for a short period of time.
- **D–E:** The level is quickly lowered in order to recover.
- **E–F:** The intensity is increased to the starting level.
- **F:** The process repeats itself.

Because of the high-intensity levels associated with interval and fartlek training, a higher degree of physical stress is placed on the structures of the body, especially at the joints. It is advisable for an individual to have an adequate cardiovascular base of fitness before undertaking this type of exercise. As all of the energy systems in the body are used during this type of training (see Chapter 6), careful planning is needed to target the systems so that the individual can achieve his or her goals. The following points should be considered:

1. The current fitness level of the individual
2. The fitness goals of the individual
3. The energy systems applicable to the goals identified
4. The duration and intensity of the build-up to the required level
5. The duration and intensity of recovery periods
6. The duration and intensity of the normal work periods
7. The number of repetitions of each cycle (overall duration).

NEED TO KNOW

Although constant rhythmic exercise is preferred by the ACSM, sports such as tennis and netball can be used in the cardiovascular conditioning phase.

Cool-down following a cardiovascular workout

The *cool-down* is sometimes referred to as a *warm-down* and these two terms can be used interchangeably. Due to the increased heart rate of the cardiovascular part of the session, individuals need to take time to gradually reduce the heart rate and blood pressure to near resting levels. This is known as the cool-down.

The ACSM recommends a period of approximately 5–10 minutes for this part of the exercise session. Individuals can use the same type of cardiovascular equipment used in the warm-up and cardiovascular endurance sessions to achieve this, but at a level that gradually reduces in intensity. In general terms, the cool-down should help to:

1. Disperse lactic acid
2. Prevent blood pooling
3. Return the body systems to normal levels
4. Assist in maintaining venous return

5. Reduce the potential for hypotension and dizziness
6. Help to dissipate body heat.

NEED TO KNOW

As a general guide, the intensity levels of the exercise should be reduced gradually throughout the cool-down until the heart rate is below 100 bpm.

Cool-down guidelines

- Reduce the level of intensity gradually
- Elicit feedback from participants on the level of intensity
- Be in a position to observe all participants
- Stretches can be included on the move if the client is balanced.

Resistance training

Resistance training can be performed using different forms of exercise, such as resistance machines, free weights and body-weight exercises. Depending on the facility, a large range of resistance machines and free weights will be available. Prior to working with clients at a new facility, instructors should familiarise themselves with the machines when working at a new facility. The resistance training part of the session should start with a warm-up and finish with a cool-down.

Benefits of resistance training

Many benefits are associated with resistance training, depending on the intensity of the resistance, the number of sets and repetitions performed, the rest periods and many other variables. Common benefits include:

1. Reduced risk of osteoporosis
2. Increase in muscle mass
3. Increase in bone mass
4. Increase in glucose tolerance
5. Increased joint integrity
6. Reduced back pain
7. Improved posture
8. Reduction of hypertension
9. Reduced risk of diabetes
10. Increased strength of connective tissue.

Warm-up for resistance training

It is not advisable to perform any muscular contractions against a resistance until the muscle or muscle groups have been prepared. This can be done by performing a number of contractions using a lighter weight than prescribed for each resistance exercise in the programme.

Main activity

Prior to designing an exercise programme that includes resistance training, it is necessary to establish the number of repetitions to be performed during the training session. This can be done either during the individual's induction or during the first training session. For example, if an individual decides to perform 10 repetitions, he or she needs to find a weight that they can lift successfully 10 times but fail on the 11th repetition. If the individual can perform more than 10 repetitions easily, the weight should be increased; if the individual cannot perform 10 repetitions, the weight should be decreased. This is a trial and error method that becomes easier to administer as the instructor gains experience.

The resistance exercise continuum

Common goals for a resistance training programme include muscular strength, endurance, hypertrophy and power. Training

Fig. 13.3 **The resistance exercise continuum**

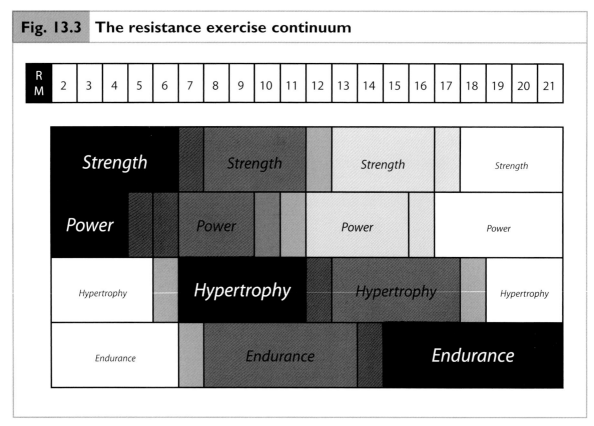

Adapted from Baechle and Earle 2000 (Increasing darkness of colour and increasing font size correspond to increased adaptation for the relevant goal at the repetition maximum).

programmes are normally devised in relation to the specific goal, but can differ depending on the level of knowledge and experience of the individual. Although there is no such thing as an optimum programme for muscular strength, endurance, hypertrophy or power gains due to the many variables that can affect the nature of a resistance training programme, there is a general and commonly used guide that shows the intensity required to elicit specific gains. This is known as the *resistance exercise continuum* (see Fig. 13.3).

In simple terms, to elicit strength gains it is logical to train with heavy loads, so the number of repetitions performed will be low. If, on the other hand, muscular endurance is the goal, it is logical to train with lighter loads and therefore perform a higher number of repetitions.

Depending on the outcome goal (strength, endurance, power or hypertrophy), a certain range of repetitions is recommended to elicit the appropriate adaptation, as can be seen in Fig. 13.3. This range is not exact and there is a certain degree of overlap due to the many variables that can affect adaptation to the specific training. The amount of weight (intensity) to be used can be based on a percentage of the individual's 1RM.

NEED TO KNOW

Research has found little difference, in terms of adaptation, between single-set and multiple-set resistance training programmes.

Free weights versus resistance machines

One of the current anecdotal debates within the health and fitness industry is whether to advocate free-weight exercises, resistance-machine exercises or both. Resistance machines vary greatly between manufacturers with respect to ergonomic design, range of adjustment and planes of movement, so it is impossible to advocate one method of resistance training over another. The advantages and disadvantages of both resistance machines and free weights must be taken into account on an individual basis (see Table 13.1). It is the instructor's responsibility to advise individuals of the benefits of both methods of resistance training and to take into account the individual's preference before designing an exercise programme.

Table 13.1	Advantages and disadvantages of different types of resistance training	
	Advantages	Disadvantages
Free weights	• Many exercises can be performed with limited equipment. • Uses synergists and fixators in a functional isotonic way. • Full range of motion is available. • Less expensive compared to machines. • Relatively portable.	• More instruction required for safety and correct technique. • Often require a training partner for safety purposes. • Do not always appeal to a broad range of users.
Resistance machines	• Relatively easy to learn and therefore to instruct. • The weight selected does not need to be calculated. • The weight setting can be changed easily.	• The plane of motion is set by the machine, which is not functional. • Can sometimes limit range of motion. • Seated positions do not replicate most functional movements. • Seat supports negate the use of core stabilisers. • Lack of synergist and fixator use. • Relatively expensive compared to free weights.

Structure of the resistance training session

Regardless of whether resistance machines, free weights or both are incorporated into a training programme, within each training session the larger muscle groups should be exercised before the smaller muscle groups. This is to prevent the smaller muscle groups becoming fatigued and affecting the exercises in which they assist the larger muscle groups. For example, if the tricep muscles were exercised to fatigue before the bench press was performed, the individual would achieve a lower than normal weight, as the tricep muscles assist the pectorals in this exercise.

Cool-down following resistance training

The requirements of a cool-down following resistance training are similar to those following cardiovascular training. At the end of each exercise, the individual should perform several repetitions of the same exercise using a lighter weight than that used in the main activity.

Flexibility training

Flexibility is the range of possible movement in a joint. Flexibility exercises can be performed prior to the main cardio session after the warm-up or at the end of the cool-down, depending on preference. The ACSM guidelines for stretching do not state when the exercises should be carried out, only that they should be performed a specific number of times per week at a certain intensity (2–4 reps of 15–30 seconds). If stretches are performed prior to the conditioning phase, they are known as *pre-stretches*, and if they are performed after the conditioning phase, they are known as *post-stretches*. The actual stretches performed are the same; it is just the name that is different.

The stretching exercises included within each exercise session should be related to the specific muscle groups that are going to be or were used during the session. Many stretches are in use throughout the health and fitness industry and the type of stretch employed can depend on several factors, including the preference of the instructor who is designing the exercise programme. However, certain stretches can place unnecessary strain on particular joints. These stretches are known as *contra-indicated* stretches and should be avoided. Table 13.2 describes some typical stretches used in the health and fitness industry. For the purpose of this book, however, the focus will be upon stretches that are not considered to be contra-indicated.

As with the other components of health-related physical fitness, it is essential that the instructor performs the correct technique when demonstrating any stretches in order for the client to copy.

TASK

List the components of an exercise session and briefly outline the ACSM recommendations relating to each component.

Periodisation

The term *periodisation* is used in both sport and health and fitness. It relates to programme design and the process of manipulation of a programme of exercise at regular intervals, known as cycles. Although periodisation is used predominantly by athletes in order to organise their training programmes so that they 'peak' at

Table 13.2 Typical stretches

Muscles stretched	Key points	Demonstration
• Pectoralis major • Anterior deltoid	1. Stand with your feet hip-width apart. 2. Clasp your hands behind your back. 3. Straighten your arms. 4. Raise your arms until you feel tension. 5. Maintain neutral spine.	
• Trapezius • Latissimus dorsi • Posteiror deltoid • Bicep brach	1. Stand with your feet hip-width apart. 2. Clasp your hands in front of you. 3. Straighten your arms away from your body. 4. Separate the scapula by pushing your shoulders forward.	

Table 13.2	Typical stretches cont.	
Muscles stretched	Key points	Demonstration
• Triceps	1. Stand with your feet hip-width apart. 2. Raise one elbow above your head. 3. Reach towards the opposite scapula. 4. Increase the stretch by pushing your elbow with the opposite hand.	
• Hip flexors	1. Adopt the lunge position. 2. Lower the hips forward and down. 3. Keep your body upright. 4. Keep your front foot flat.	

Table 13.2	Typical stretches cont.	
Muscles stretched	Key points	Demonstration
• Quadriceps	1. Clasp the front of your foot. 2. Take your heel towards your bottom. 3. Keep your knees almost together. 4. Maintain neutral spine.	
• Hamstrings	1. Sit on the floor with neutral spine. 2. Place the heel of one foot on the inside of the opposite knee. 3. Lean forward from the waist. 4. Maintain neutral spine.	

Table 13.2   Typical stretches cont.

Muscles stretched	Key points	Demonstration
• Hip adductors	1. Sit on the floor with your legs wide apart. 2. Lean to one side, facing forward. 3. Bend the knee of the side to which you are leaning. 4. Keep the opposite leg straight.	
• Hip abductors	1. Sit on the floor with one leg out straight in front of you. 2. Cross the opposite leg over the straight leg. 3. Sit upright and hug your knee to your chest.	

competition times, it is also used in the health and fitness industry as a goal-setting tool: the regular manipulation of an exercise programme is thought to elicit optimal gains in one or more of the components of fitness.

In order to achieve this, it is common to monitor ongoing performance so that the programme can be adjusted accordingly depending on the nature of the results. The programme can be organised into intervals known as cycles. Each type of cycle has a different time allocation:

- **Microcycle:** this is the shortest period of training within an exercise programme and normally refers to the number of training sessions in a seven-day period (that is, short-term planning). Obviously, any goals within such a short period of time need to be achievable in relation to the individual.
- **Mesocycle:** this is a repeating series of microcycles over a period of several weeks (that is, medium-term planning). The goals in a mesocycle should be achievable yet flexible, as they can be manipulated following analysis of the microcycles within it.
- **Macrocycle:** this is a series of mesocycles, normally over a period of a few months to several years (that is, long-term planning). Information gathered from microcycles and mesocycles can be used to confirm or readjust the long-term goals of the macrocycle.

Each microcycle contributes to the goals of the mesocycles, which in turn will contribute to the goals of the overall macrocycle. It is important that the instructor constantly revises the goals of each cycle due to the constant interaction of one cycle on another. Planning a programme of exercise using periodised cycles can be useful as it can give individual short-, medium- and long-term goals (see Chapter 12). This has been shown to have a positive effect on adherence

to exercise, not only for beginners but for regular exercisers as well. When designing an exercise programme, it is recommended that it is recorded simply and accurately, so that the individual can use it as a reference during exercise sessions. There are many ways of designing a periodised exercise programme but one of the more common methods is that of the step-loading model.

The step-loading method

Simple progressive overload training programmes are often thought to be boring and repetitive for the individual, as well as leading to staleness and increasing the risk of repetitive loading injuries. This is the opposite case with the step-loading programmes, which are thought to decrease the risk of repetitive injuries. Step-loading models normally include 2 or 3 short cycles (microcycles) of increases in intensity followed by a short cycle of decreased intensity (similar in intensity to the second cycle) before repeating the process again. The simple model shown in Fig. 13.4 can relate to either cardiovascular or resistance training programmes.

It can be seen in the example of a step loading model that short cycles of specific intensities can be performed in sequence.

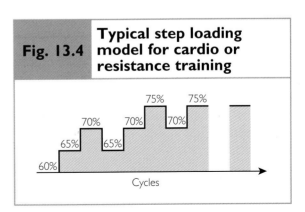

Fig. 13.4 Typical step loading model for cardio or resistance training

60% 65% 70% 65% 70% 75% 70% 75%

Cycles

Again, the intensities are just examples which depend on many variables relating to the individual and the event that they are training for. The step loading model can also be thought of in terms of low, moderate and high intensity cycles that increase in intensity when repeated. Quite often these cycles are a week long where the moderate training intensity week is usually representative of an average training week and the low and high intensity weeks are adjusted to this level.

Recording exercise programmes

There are many ways of recording exercise programmes, but for a session within a microcycle it is common to use a session card (see Fig. 13.5) that provides information relating to one session only. A typical session card contains all the information relevant to the individual performing the exercise, as well as information regarding the specific exercise plan. Be aware that information contained on a session card can be confidential so must be treated as such.

Induction sessions

The term *induction* is used to describe the process of the instructor explaining to the client the details and requirements of the exercise session in relation to their specific programme, and showing them how the exercise session will be carried out in the environment they are going to use. For example, inductions that take place in a gym aim to familiarise the client with the operation of the equipment and the performance of the exercises in relation to the

session. Therefore, as well as explaining how to operate any equipment, the induction should take the client through each component of the exercise session in turn (warm-up, cardio, cool-down, resistance and flexibility) to make sure they understand and practise each component. This will also give the instructor the opportunity to identify client training intensities in relation to cardiovascular and resistance equipment settings.

Client induction sessions are normally carried out following a successful client screening session (see Chapter 11) in which it was agreed that the client could begin a programme of exercise. There are no specific guidelines relating to client induction procedures, which is one of the reasons why all health and fitness facilities tend to have their own methods for client induction. However, regardless of the method used for induction sessions, common guidelines can be applied. These guidelines relate to a client induction for the cardiovascular, resistance and flexibility components of the session to be performed.

Warm-up, cardio and cool-down induction

The facility in which the instructor is working will determine the type of cardiovascular machines available. When working at a new facility, instructors are advised to familiarise themselves with the machines prior to inducting individuals.

Before individuals begin a programme of exercise, they need to be given an induction relating to their specific exercise programme, starting with the first session. Following an explanation of the controls of the cardiovascular machines, it is usual for the instructor to take the individual through their training session in order to establish cardiovascular intensity levels for the warm-up, main activity and cool-down. There are many methods of inducting individuals on cardiovascular machines depending on the

Fig. 13.5   **Example session plan template**

SESSION PLAN: Number: Page:

Instructor name: Client name: Ability level:

Objectives:

Duration (reps, seconds, circuits, etc.)	Exercises (name muscles used and draw diagrams where needed)	Equipment	Sets	Intensity (speed, rpm, weight, level)	Alternative and progression (and coaching points)

First Aid point: Tel:

Resources: Music:

individual instructor's preference. However, in order to be consistent in the delivery, it is advisable to use a logical approach such as the acronym IDEA, which can be used regardless of the cardiovascular machine being used:

I   Introduce the exercise.
D   Demonstrate the correct technique.
E   Explain the exercise using minimal coaching points.
A   Activity: observe the client doing the activity on the machine.

It is important that instructors use correct technique when demonstrating so that the individual does not copy 'bad' technique. As the visual demonstration will provide a great deal of information for the individual, the verbal information that supplements this can be kept to a minimum. When the individual is using the machine, the instructor should maintain a dialogue in order to give them relevant information on performance and technique. The instructor should then aim to identify the suitable training intensity.

Even though a vast range of cardiovascular training equipment is available, there are many common guidelines that can be employed when using the equipment (see Table 13.3).

The treadmill can be used for both walking and running, but is associated with greater impact on the joints than other cardiovascular machines. The cycle doesn't involve any impact, so can be used for individuals who need to

Table 13.3	Guidelines for cardiovascular equipment
Treadmill	**Foot action:** A heel–toe action should be encouraged when walking or jogging, as this will help to absorb the shock of impact. At speeds around 8 mph, the client should be encouraged to use a mid-foot strike, as this will help to eliminate the braking effect.
	Arm action: The most efficient way to swing the arms is with a 90-degree angle at the elbows and with the arms swinging close to the side of the body. Try to keep the shoulders relaxed at all times.
	Posture: Encourage the client to maintain a neutral spine with only a slight forward lean, which should increase slightly as the treadmill is inclined.
Cycle	**Seat height:** As the seat height can affect the range of motion and speed of the legs, it is important to make sure that the seat is level with the hip joint of the client when standing next to the cycle. With the client on the cycle and the feet flat in the pedals, the knee should have a slight bend at the furthest point of the rotation.
	Pedal speed (cadence): Actual pedal speed depends on the preference of the client. Most people prefer to pedal between 50 and 80 rpm, although this can increase during bouts of high intensity.
	Posture: Encourage an upright posture with neutral spine at all times. If using a recumbent cycle, encourage clients not to press their back flat into the seat and to try to maintain a neutral spine.

Table 13.3	Guidelines for cardiovascular equipment cont.
Stepper	**Range of motion:** With the whole of the foot placed on the step, encourage a full range of motion that is just before the end range of the machine. **Action:** As the leg raises during the stepping, the heel of the same leg should raise slightly off the pedal and return to the pedal as the leg goes down. **Speed:** Select a speed that is comfortable for the client. As the level on the step machine is increased, the resistance of the pedals will decrease, which means that the client will need to increase the speed. **Posture:** Encourage the client to hold the handles just to the side of the body rather than out in front. This will enable the client to maintain an upright posture with neutral spine.
Rower	**Start position (catch):** With the feet secured in the straps and the knees bent, hold the handle with a pronated grip (overhand) with the arms out straight and a slight bend at the elbows. Keep the wrists straight. The back should be in an upright neutral position. **Drive:** Initiate the drive phase with the legs pushing out. When the legs are almost at full stretch, pull the handle into the abdomen area. **Recovery:** The arms must extend fully before the legs bend to allow the body to come back to the start position. The recovery phase should be twice as long as the drive phase.

reduce the amount of impact to the joints, such as those with obesity or arthritis. As with the treadmill, the cycle can be used for either aerobic or anaerobic conditioning, depending on the intensity of the exercise. Stepping and rowing are also non-impact machines that can be used for individuals wishing to avoid any impact on the joints, but it is important to remember that rowing can place a greater amount of stress on the lower back than other methods of cardiovascular exercise.

It is also recommended that information regarding health and safety is given to the individual during the induction session. Fire exits and emergency procedures can be pointed out, as well as water and toilet facilities. The individual should also be made aware that they should terminate exercise at any time should they feel unwell or unable to continue.

NEED TO KNOW

The loss of balance that sometimes occurs when a treadmill comes to a stop is due to confusion in the brain, as the brain is used to objects in the distance becoming nearer when moving forward.

Resistance induction

Most beginners to resistance training are unfamiliar with the operation of resistance machines and free weights. It is therefore important to give clear explanations of how to operate resistance machines and the techniques involved in resistance training before the individual begins an exercise programme.

As with the cardio induction, the instructor usually takes the individual through their resistance training session in order to establish intensity levels for the warm-up, main activity and cool-down. There are many methods of inducting individuals in relation to resistance training, depending on the individual instructor's preference. However, in order to be consistent in the delivery, it is advisable to use a logical approach such as the NAMSIT method:

N	Name the machine or exercise
A	Area of the body working
M	Muscle group name
S	Silent demonstration
I	Instruct client to try
T	Teach the client

This approach can be used regardless of the resistance machine being used. It is important that instructors use good technique when demonstrating to prevent the individual copying 'bad' technique.

As with the cardiovascular demonstration, the visual demonstration for resistance exercises will provide a lot of information, so supplementary verbal information should be kept to a minimum.

When the individual is using the machine, the instructor should maintain a dialogue in order to give relevant information on performance and technique. The instructor should then aim to identify the suitable training intensity required for each resistance exercise.

Flexibility induction

As with any other part of the induction it is important that the instructor provides a technically correct demonstration of all the stretches included in the exercise programme. The gym environment should have a matted area for stretching. It is logical to start with standing stretches and then progress to seated stretches, in order to decrease the heart rate progressively. Once the instructor has demonstrated the stretch, the individual should perform it. The instructor should then give feedback about the individual's technique and give instructions about the intensity and duration of the stretch.

TASK

Explain the two common methods of cardiovascular and resistance training induction, referring to their acronyms.

EXAMPLE QUESTIONS

13.1 According to research what is considered to be the main factor in muscular injury prevention?

a) strength

b) muscle temperature

c) flexibility

d) stretching

13.2 In terms of cardiovascular training at the end of the warm-up, the heart rate should be at what level?

a) the heart rate is irrelevant as long as the individual is warm

b) 60% max heart rate

c) that required for the cardiovascular session to follow

d) maximum

13.3 In relation to cardio training zones, what range of heart range maximum is the 'weight management zone'?

a) 50–60%

b) 60–70%

c) 70–80%

d) 80–90%

13.4 In relation to cardio training zones, what range of heart range maximum is the 'aerobic zone'?

a) 50–60%

b) 60–70%

c) 70–80%

d) 80–90%

13.5 Which of the following are considered to be the main benefits of cardiovascular training?

a) decreased fat metabolism, increased glycogen stores, increased aerobic and anaerobic enzymes, increased number and size of mitochondria

EXAMPLE QUESTIONS cont.

b) increased fat metabolism, decreased glycogen stores, increased aerobic and anaerobic enzymes, increased number and size of mitochondria

c) increased fat metabolism, increased glycogen stores, decreased aerobic and anaerobic enzymes, increased number and size of mitochondria

d) increased fat metabolism, increased glycogen stores, increased aerobic and anaerobic enzymes, increased number and size of mitochondria

13.6 What type of training is otherwise known as 'speed play'?
a) interval
b) continuous
c) intermittent
d) Fartlek

13.7 Which cycle of periodisation is usually associated with a 7-day period?
a) minicycle
b) microcycle
c) mesocycle
d) macrocycle

13.8 Which cycle of periodisation is usually associated with a period of a few weeks?
a) minicycle
b) microcycle
c) mesocycle
d) macrocycle

13.9 Which cycle of periodisation is usually associated with a 12-month period?
a) minicycle
b) microcycle
c) mesocycle
d) macrocycle

EXAMPLE QUESTIONS cont.

13.10 The ACSM guidelines for stretching suggest holding the stretch for what period of time?
- **a)** 5–10 seconds
- **b)** 15–30 seconds
- **c)** 10–20 seconds
- **d)** 30–45 seconds

13.11 The acronym IDEA refers to what?
- **a)** induction for cardiovascular machines
- **b)** induction for resistance machines
- **c)** the screening process
- **d)** risk stratification

13.12 Which of the following cardiovascular machines is normally associated with higher impact?
- **a)** cycle
- **b)** stepper
- **c)** treadmill
- **d)** rower

Further reading

American College of Sports Medicine (2009) *ACSM Guidelines to Exercise Testing and Prescription* (8th ed.), Lippincott, Williams & Wilkins

Baechle, R.T. (2008) *Essentials of Strength Training and Conditioning* (3rd ed.), Human Kinetics

Bompa, T.O. (2009) *Periodisation Theory and Methodology of Training* (5th ed.), Human Kinetics

Bouchard, C., Shepard, R. and Stephens, T. (1994) *Physical Activity, Fitness and Health*, Human Kinetics

Howley, E.T. and Franks, B.D. (2003) *Health Fitness Instructor's Handbook* (4th ed.), Human Kinetics

Marieb, E.N. (2009) *Human Anatomy and Physiology* (8th ed.), Benjamin Cummings Publishing Company Inc.

McArdle, W.D., Katch, F.I. and Katch, V.L. (2007) *Exercise Physiology* (6th ed.), Lippincott, Williams & Wilkins

Ross, J.S. and Wilson, J.W. (2006) *Anatomy and Physiology in Health and Illness* (10th ed.), Churchill Livingstone

Sewell, D., Watkins, P. and Griffin, M. (2005) *Sport and Exercise Science: An Introduction*, Hodder Arnold

Stratton, G., Jones, M., Fox, K.R., Tolfrey, K., Harris, J., Maffulli, N., Lee, M. and Frostick, S.P. (2004) 'BASES position statement on guidelines for resistance exercise in young people', *Journal of Sports Sciences*, 22(4): 383–390

Tortora, G.J. and Grabowski, S.R. (2005) *Principles of Anatomy and Physiology* (11th ed.), Wiley

Wilmore, J.H. and Costhill, D.L. (2004) *Physiology of Sport and Exercise* (3rd ed.), Human Kinetics

NOTES

MONITORING EXERCISE INTENSITY 14

OBJECTIVES

After completing this chapter, you will be able to:

1 List and describe the cardiovascular training zones associated with the health and fitness industry.

2 Explain the various methods of monitoring cardiovascular and resistance exercise intensity.

3 Calculate percentages of heart rate maximum.

Level 2: Instructing Exercise and Fitness Knowledge

Basic Anatomy and Physiology
- Exercises that are safe and appropriate for participants.
- How to plan to use a range of cardiovascular and resistance machines and weights.

Level 3: Instructing Physical Activity and Exercise Knowledge

Energy Systems and Components of Fitness
- Heart-rate training zones
- METS
- Monitoring exercise intensity:
  - RPE, talk test, lactic testing, heart rate monitoring
  - Benefits and limitations of each method

Introduction

This chapter deals with common methods of prescribing and monitoring exercise intensity employed within the health and fitness industry in relation to guidelines within the National Occupational Standards for health and fitness. Level 2 and 3 instructors should be able to list the common methods of monitoring cardiovascular and resistance exercise intensity and explain each within the context of the health and fitness industry.

Other chapters in the book provide information regarding the practical application of the theoretical content which, along with the information covered in this chapter, will provide instructors with the understanding and ability to design appropriate exercise programmes for apparently healthy individuals, in line with current guidelines for exercise.

Exercise intensity

Intensity refers to the difficulty level of a particular exercise or, in simple terms, how hard the exercise feels to the individual. When designing an exercise programme, instructors can prescribe intensity levels that best suit the individual's goals. For example, an individual might have weight loss and toning as goals. In this case, the instructor could set cardiovascular intensity within the weight-management training zone and resistance training intensity at around 10–12 RM (see Chapter 10).

Monitoring the intensity level at which an individual is exercising can also help instructors to adjust the exercise programme accordingly. Monitoring can give the instructor information regarding fitness progression or any drop in performance that might indicate signs of overtraining, allowing him or her to use this information to make necessary adjustments to the programme.

When prescribing exercise at a specific intensity, it is useful to understand the physiology in relation to each component of fitness (see Chapter 10). Intensity levels of both cardiovascular exercise and resistance exercise can be monitored in several different ways. Monitoring intensity within a health and fitness environment is not as accurate as monitoring within a laboratory environment, but is still useful if the lack of accuracy is taken into consideration.

Monitoring cardiovascular intensity

Several methods can be used to prescribe and monitor a particular cardiovascular exercise intensity for an individual, including heart rate, metabolic equivalents, self-perception (rate of perceived exertion) and communication skills (the talk test).

Heart rate

One of the most common methods of prescribing or monitoring cardiovascular intensity is the heart rate method. As the intensity of the exercise increases, the heart rate of the individual increases in a linear fashion. It therefore follows that, as training zones are related to a percentage of maximum heart rate, the percentage of maximum heart rate that has been agreed for the exercise can be related to the goals of the individual. For example, if the individual wants to develop aerobic fitness, he or she should exercise at a heart rate level of 70–80 per cent of their maximum (the aerobic zone). This can be written as 70–80%HRM.

Two steps need to be taken in order to convert the chosen percentage of heart rate maximum into beats per minute. First, the maximum heart rate of the individual needs to be found; second, the required percentage of this maximum needs to be calculated.

Step 1: Calculating the maximum heart rate of an individual.

Maximum heart rate can be calculated by using one of two methods: one way is to carry out a maximum graded heart rate test, and the other is to use a formula for predicting maximum heart rate.

Maximum graded heart rate test

Several tests are available in which intensity is increased until the point at which there is no rise in heart rate, even though the intensity is continuing to increase. This type of test is reasonably accurate, but is not suitable for any individual who is tested within the health and fitness environment, as National Occupational Standards guidelines recommend that instructors advise exercise intensity only up to a maximum of 90 per cent of heart rate maximum.

Predicted maximum heart rate

As an alternative to a maximum graded heart rate test, the following formula can be used to predict maximum heart rate:

$$\text{Maximum Heart Rate} = 220 - \text{age}$$

For example, a 23-year-old person would have a predicted maximum heart rate of 197 bpm ($220 - 23 = 197$) and a 45-year-old person would have a predicted maximum heart rate of 175 bpm ($220 - 45$). Even though there are errors associated with this method of estimating maximum heart rate (there can be an error of plus or minus 12 bpm using this method), it is commonly used and is suitable for the health and fitness industry.

Step 2: Calculating the percentage of the maximum heart rate in bpm

Once the maximum heart rate has been established, it is possible to calculate the percentage of heart rate maximum that is required for the individual in beats per minute (bpm): the maximum heart rate for the individual is multiplied by the chosen percentage. For instance, a 32-year-old individual needs to perform the exercise at 70–80 per cent of maximum heart rate (the aerobic zone). The instructor should calculate the individual's training intensity heart rates at 70 and 80 per cent of maximum as follows:

1. Predicted maximum heart rate for the individual is 220 – age (32) = 188 bpm
2. 70 per cent of maximum (188 bpm) = 188/100 × 70 = 131 bpm
3. 80 per cent of maximum (188 bpm) = (188/100 × 80) = 150 bpm

Note: Round the answer to the nearest whole number.

Therefore, in order to exercise at the desired intensity, the individual would need to keep his or her heart rate between 131 bpm and 150 bpm. Over a period of time, if the individual could maintain this heart rate but at an increased speed, this would indicate that the individual was becoming fitter. This is one method of monitoring cardiovascular fitness.

Metabolic equivalents (METs)

The intensity of an exercise can be linked to the amount of energy expended by the individual: the greater the intensity level of the exercise, the greater the energy expenditure required to sustain that level. A *metabolic equivalent* or *MET* is a way of expressing expenditure in either calories (kcal) or volume of oxygen (VO_2). The resting value of 1 MET is expressed as follows:

$$1 \text{ MET} = 3.5 \text{ mlO}_2.\text{kg}^{-1}\text{min}^{-1} \text{ or } 1\text{kcal.kg}^{-1}\text{hr}^{-1}$$

It follows that an exercise that requires four times as much energy than that used at rest would have a value of 4 METs and an exercise that requires 10 times as much would have a value of 10 METs, and so on. Even though MET values are commonly shown on cardiovascular machines, the use of metabolic equivalents seems to be restricted to medical use for exercise

Table 14.1 Metabolic equivalents for various activities

Activities between 3 and 6 METs	Activities of more than 6 METs
Housework:	**Housework:**
Polishing	Any heavy housework
Cleaning windows	Any heavy gardening
Making beds	
Mopping floors	**Activities:**
Vacuuming	Jogging
Hanging washing	Running
Sweeping	Brisk cycling
Gardening – light work	Brisk swimming
	Wheeling in wheelchair
Activities:	High-impact aerobics
Slow walking	Martial arts
Brisk walking	Circuit training
Slow cycling	Skipping
Slow swimming	
Skating	**Sports:**
Gentle aerobics	Dancing
Yoga	Tennis
Dancing (ballroom, etc.)	Horse riding
Golf	Squash
Table tennis	Basketball
	Football
Sports:	Gymnastics
Fencing	Fencing
Archery	Skiing
Cricket	Rugby
	Netball
	Boxing

prescription. If the machines used do not display MET values, there are many published tables that estimate them for a range of activities (see Table 14.1). These activities can extend to household chores and outdoor activities as well as fitness facility activities.

Note: This table has been adapted from a variety of sources and should be used as an approximation of metabolic equivalent values related to various activities.

As METs have a value expressed in calories, if the weight of the individual is known, then the amount of calories expended during a particular exercise can also be calculated. Take, for example, a 75 kg person exercising at 10 METs for one hour:

10 METs = 10 kcals per kilo of bodyweight every hour, and 10 (kcals) × 75 (kg) = 750. Therefore, this person would expend 750 kcals.

NEED TO KNOW

Any activities between 3 and 6 METs are considered moderate-intensity physical activity. Any activities greater than 6 METs are considered vigorous-intensity physical activity.

Rate of perceived exertion (RPE)

Another method of setting and monitoring the appropriate exercise intensity for an individual is to use the *rate of perceived exertion* (*RPE*) scale (see Table 14.2), which was first introduced by Dr Gunnar Borg and is sometimes known as the Borg scale.

The RPE scale is a method of measuring the subjective feelings of an individual during exercise. The individual's perception of the level of difficulty during cardiovascular exercise has been found to correlate very strongly with heart rate. For this reason, the RPE scale is widely used as an alternative to heart rate.

Two different scales are commonly used: the 6–20 scale and the revised 0–10+ scale, also known as the *category ratio* or *CR-10 scale*. The individual is shown the scale during exercise and asked how he or she feels compared to the words on the scale. This perception is then used to estimate either the percentage of heart rate maximum or the heart rate. For example, if the individual states that the exercise feels 'somewhat hard', this equates to level 13 on the 6–20 scale, which corresponds to approximately 130 bpm or 70 per cent of MHR. Depending on the goals of the individual, the instructor can recommend an RPE level at which to exercise without the need to monitor heart rate.

Even though the subjective perception of exercise intensity correlates well with heart rate, it is important to note that various individuals carrying out exactly the same exercise session might report different levels of RPE. There are many factors that could affect this perception rating, such as fitness levels, exercise familiarity and illness.

NEED TO KNOW

Research has shown that perception rating on the 6–20 scale correlates closely with heart rate: for example, a 'very light' rating equates to 9 on the scale, which would be a heart rate of approximately 90 bpm.

Talk test

Although the talk test is not a particularly scientific method of determining cardiovascular exercise intensity, it can be used as an alternative to heart rate, METs or RPE due to the ease of administration. The talk test is simply a matter of talking to the individual during exercise and gauging the level of intensity from the response of the individual. If the individual is able to carry out a normal conversation, this usually indicates that he or she is in either the weight-management zone or the lower end of the aerobic zone.

Table 14.2	Rate of perceived exertion (Borg) scale	
6–20 scale	0–10 scale	Estimate of %MHR
6	0 Nothing at all	
7 Very, very light	0.3	
8	0.5 Extremely weak	50%
9 very light	0.7	55%
10	1 Very weak	60%
11 Fairly light	1.5	65%
12	2 Weak	70%
13 Somewhat hard	2.5	75%
14	3 Moderate	80%
15 Hard	4	85%
16	5 Strong	88%
17 Very hard	6	92%
18	7 Very strong	96%
19 Very, very hard	8	98%
20	9	100%
	10 Extremely strong	
	11	
	Absolute maximum	

Adapted from *ACSM Guidelines for Exercise Testing and Prescription* and Lippincott, Williams & Wilkins (2006).

If the individual becomes breathless and has difficulty maintaining a normal conversation, this usually means he or she is in the anaerobic zone. The instructor can then adjust the level of intensity accordingly, depending on the goal of the exercise session.

Once the required level of intensity of a cardiovascular exercise session has been attained using the talk test method, the instructor can empower the individual to take responsibility for maintaining that level in subsequent exercise sessions. The individual should be informed that they can progress by increasing the intensity of the exercise, as long as they are still able to carry out a normal conversation.

TASK

 List the methods of monitoring cardiovascular intensity and briefly describe how each method is used.

Monitoring resistance intensity

When prescribing the intensity of a resistance exercise (how heavy the weight should be), the instructor can use a percentage of the maximum capability of that individual, known as 1 repetition maximum or 1RM. However, one disadvantage of this method is that the maximum capability of the individual must be found before a percentage of this can be calculated. As the individual would have to perform to maximum capability, the risk of injury would be high and not in line with recommended guidelines.

An easier method would be to use a multiple of the repetition maximum, such as 10RM or 15RM, which means the maximum weight the individual can lift 10 or 15 times respectively. The ACSM guidelines for strength and endurance are given in multiples of RM. For example, in order to gain strength it is recommended that an individual performs resistance exercise using weights within the range of 8–12RM, and to improve endurance using weights within the range of 10–15RM. Research has shown that the multiple of repetition maximum correlates to a percentage of the maximum capability (see Table 14.3).

Calculating repetition maximum

When trying to establish the amount of weight an individual can lift for a specific number of repetitions (repetition maximum), a certain procedure should be used to ensure that the individual is sufficiently warmed in order to minimise the risk of injury. If the instructor and the individual have agreed that an intensity of 12RM is going to be used for a particular

Table 14.3	Repetition maximum compared to percentage of maximum capability
Repetition maximum	% of maximum capability
1	100.0
2	93.5
3	91.0
4	88.5
5	86.0
6	83.5
7	81.0
8	78.5
9	76.0

Adapted from Baechle (2000).

exercise, the individual should first perform 12 repetitions of a known light weight. Then add more weight depending on the ease of the first set and have the individual perform another 12 repetitions. Repeat this process until the individual can perform 12 repetitions only, and not 13. Ensure that sufficient rest is given between sets to recover: two to three minutes should be sufficient. The final weight (or load) that the individual could lift 12 times (but fail on the 13th) is the 12RM for that particular exercise. This process should then be repeated for all of the exercises in the resistance training programme.

For progression purposes (and assuming that the multiple repetition maximum chosen is to remain constant), when the individual is capable of comfortably performing the chosen repetition maximum, the weight can be increased by a small amount. If the individual cannot perform the number of chosen repetitions at the increased weight, he or she must revert to the original weight. This type of in-built progression is easy to implement and, as such, the instructor should empower the individual to take control of monitoring their own progression.

TASK

Briefly describe the term *repetition maximum* and explain how it is used to determine the intensity of the resistance exercise to be performed.

EXAMPLE QUESTIONS

14.1 What is the formula for predicted maximum heart rate?
a) 200 - age
b) 210 - age
c) 220 - age
d) 230 - age

14.2 True or false? Predicted maximum heart rate can have an error of up to plus or minus 12 beats per minute.

True ☐   False ☐

14.3 True or false? A graded maximum heart rate test should be used on all individuals to find their maximum heart rate.

True ☐   False ☐

14.4 What is the predicted maximum heart rate for a 29 year old person?
a) 201 bpm
b) 191 bpm
c) 189 bpm
d) 199 bpm

14.5 What is 70% of predicted maximum heart rate for a 40-year-old person?
a) 106 bpm
b) 116 bpm
c) 126 bpm
d) 136 bpm

14.6 What is 80% of predicted maximum heart rate for a 20-year-old person?
a) 160 bpm
b) 170 bpm
c) 150 bpm
d) 180 bpm

EXAMPLE QUESTIONS cont.

14.7 What is 55% of predicted maximum heart rate for a 31-year-old person (round up)?
a) 101 bpm
b) 124 bpm
c) 114 bpm
d) 104 bpm

14.8 What is the equivalent value of 2 MET?
a) 3.5 $mlO_2.kg^{-1}min^{-1}$
b) 5 $mlO_2.kg^{-1}min^{-1}$
c) 7 $mlO_2.kg^{-1}min^{-1}$
d) 9.5 $mlO_2.kg^{-1}min^{-1}$

14.9 What is the equivalent value of 1 MET?
a) 1.0 $kcal.kg^{-1}hr^{-1}$
b) 1.5 $kcal.kg^{-1}hr^{-1}$
c) 2.0 $kcal.kg^{-1}hr^{-1}$
d) 2.5 $kcal.kg^{-1}hr^{-1}$

14.10 How many kilocalories would an 80kg person expend in 30 minutes doing an exercise valued at 5 METs?
a) 100
b) 200
c) 300
d) 400

14.11 How many kilocalories would an 60kg person expend in 2 hours and 30 minutes doing an exercise valued at 4 METs?
a) 400
b) 500
c) 600
d) 700

EXAMPLE QUESTIONS cont.

14.12 Which of the following statements is most accurate in regards to the definition of 12RM?

a) A weight that can be easily lifted 12 times

b) A weight at which the performer fails on the 12th repetition

c) A weight that can be lifted at least 12 times

d) A weight that can be lifted 12 times and not 13 times

Further reading

American College of Sports Medicine (2009) *ACSM Guidelines to Exercise Testing and Prescription* (8th ed.), Lippincott, Williams & Wilkins

Baechle, R.T. (2008) *Essentials of Strength Training and Conditioning* (3rd ed.), Human Kinetics

Bouchard, C., Shepard, R. and Stephens, T. (1994) *Physical Activity, Fitness and Health*, Human Kinetics

Howley, E.T. and Franks, B.D. (2003) *Health Fitness Instructor's Handbook* (4th ed.), Human Kinetics

Marieb, E.N. (2009) *Human Anatomy and Physiology* (8th ed.), Benjamin Cummings Publishing Company Inc.

McArdle, W.D., Katch, F.I. and Katch, V.L. (2007) *Exercise Physiology* (6th ed.), Lippincott, Williams & Wilkins

Ross, J.S. and Wilson, J.W. (2006) *Anatomy and Physiology in Health and Illness* (10th ed.), Churchill Livingstone

Sewell, D., Watkins, P. and Griffin, M. (2005) *Sport and Exercise Science: An Introduction*, Hodder Arnold

Tortora, G.J. and Grabowski, S.R. (2005) *Principles of Anatomy and Physiology* (11th ed.), Wiley

Wilmore, J. H. and Costhill, D. L. (2004) *Physiology of Sport and Exercise* (3rd ed.), Human Kinetics

NOTES

FREE-WEIGHT AND RESISTANCE MACHINE EXERCISES

15

OBJECTIVES

After completing this chapter, the reader should be able to:

1 List and describe common free-weight and resistance machine exercises associated with the health and fitness industry.

2 Describe how each exercise is carried out in terms of technique.

3 List the major muscles and synergists responsible for the exercises.

4 Give alternatives for each exercise.

Level 2: Instructing Exercise and Fitness Knowledge

Basic Anatomy and Physiology

- Exercises that are safe and appropriate for participants.

- How to plan to use a range of cardiovascular and resistance machines, weights.

- The effect of speed on posture, alignment and intensity.

- The effect of levers, gravity and resistance on the exercise.

- A range of resistance machines, weights, barbells, dumbbells, collars, benches, protective floor mats.

- The safe storage of free-weight equipment.

- Safe manual handling techniques.

Introduction

This chapter deals with common free-weight and resistance machine exercises employed within the health and fitness industry. Within the National Occupational Standards framework, Level 2 and 3 instructors should be able to list the common resistance exercises and the major muscles used in each. Instructors should also be able to describe how to perform and give alternatives to each exercise.

This chapter builds upon the information in other chapters of this book, regarding the practical application of the theoretical content, to provide the instructor with an understanding of the correct performance technique associated with a range of free-weight and resistance machine exercises.

Free-weight and resistance exercises

The choice of performing resistance exercises using free-weights or machines is an individual preference. However, there are several issues that are common within the health and fitness environment (see Table 15.1).

The examples of free-weight and resistance machine exercises given in this chapter are typical of those used by beginners to this type of training. There are many other exercises common to the health and fitness environment, which can be considered to be more advanced, or for those with at least several months experience of weight training. It is crucial that all beginners to resistance exercises are shown the correct technique in a demonstration prior to performing the exercise themselves. Beginners must also be shown safety-related points, such as how to attach collars to weight lifting bars, how to pick up and return free-weights from their storage racks and how to keep the exercise area clear of obstructions. As research is sparse in relation to musculoskeletal injury as a consequence of resistance training, the following examples describe how to perform each exercise with what is considered to be safe technique within the health and fitness industry. The major and synergistic muscles (see Chapter 4) for each exercise are also listed along with alternatives for each exercise that involve the same muscle groups.

Table 15.1	Health and fitness issues
Issue	Comment
Type of equipment	**Barbell** A long bar with weights attached at either end for use with both hands. **Dumbbell** A small bar with weights attached at either end for use with one hand only. **Collars** These are used on barbells and dumbbells to prevent the weights coming off. They must be used at all times with free-weights. **Benches** Make sure benches are robust enough to use with free-weights. **Floor mats** These are recommended in the area where free-weights are used to prevent damage to the floor and the weights.

Table 15.1	Health and fitness issues cont.
Speed of execution	All exercises must be performed under control so that muscles are worked through their full range and posture is not compromised.
Range of movement	Always use the full range of movement possible for each exercise. Try to keep the repetitions continuous rather than rest at either the start or mid-point.
Breathing	A breath out is normally done prior to the exertion of the exercise. If this is confusing, just breathe normally.
Alignment	Neutral posture must be maintained during all exercises.
Storage	Return free-weights to their storage racks after use.
Handling technique	When lifting free-weights from the floor, adopt a squat position and keep the weights close to the body.
Levers	To increase the intensity of the exercise, take weights further from the body (increase lever length).
Gravity	For free-weights to be effective the weight must travel in a vertical direction.

Chest Press

Major muscles used: Pectoralis major

Synergist muscles used: Anterior deltoid, tricep, serratus anterior

Main movement: Horizontal adduction of the shoulder/extension of the elbow

- Make sure the feet are placed firmly on the ground and that the upper arms are parallel to the floor.
- The palms should be facing forwards and the hands should be directly above the elbows.
- Raise the weights in an arcing motion keeping them in line with the chest until the arms are fully extended.

Awareness points: Keep the hands directly above the elbows at all times and make sure that the wrists remain firm. Lower the weights under control until the upper arms are parallel with the floor. Maintain a normal lumbar curve at all times.

Safety point: Starting the movement with the upper arms parallel to the floor should ensure that the pectoralis major is responsible for the majority of the effort. Staring at a lower point could strain the anterior deltoid as this muscle will then be taking most of the strain in order to initiate the movement.

Alternatives: Machine Chest Press, Chest Flye, Pec Dec, Press-up.

Fig. 15.1 **(a) and (b): Chest Press**

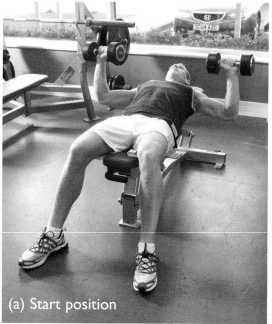

(a) Start position

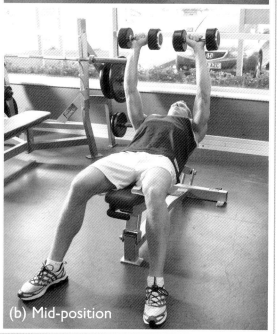

(b) Mid-position

Chest Flye

Major muscles used: Pectoralis major

Synergist muscles used: Anterior deltoid, serratus anterior

Main movement: Horizontal adduction of the shoulder

- Make sure the feet are placed firmly on the ground and that the upper arms are parallel to the floor.
- Do not extend the arms fully. Maintain a slight flexion at the elbow joint with the palms facing upwards.
- Bring the weights together in an arcing motion keeping them in line with the chest.

Awareness points: Avoid fully extending the arms at all times. Lower the weights under control until the upper arms are parallel with the floor and the hands are within peripheral vision. Maintain a normal lumbar curve at all times.

Safety point: As with all exercises, if the hands are in peripheral vision, then the risk of impingement injury at the acromion process (joint between the scapula and clavicle) is reduced.

Alternatives: Chest Press, Pec Dec, Press-up.

Fig. 15.2	(a) and (b): Chest Flye

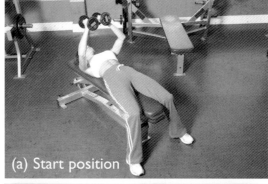
(a) Start position

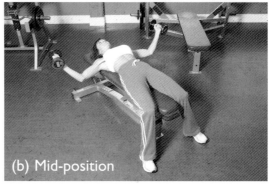
(b) Mid-position

Single Arm Row

Major muscles used: Latissimus dorsi

Synergist muscles used: Bicep brachialis, posterior deltoid

Main movement: Extension of the shoulder/ flexion of the elbow

- Adopt a kneeling position with one leg so that the hip joint of that leg is approximately 90 degrees and the supporting hand is directly below the shoulder.
- Place the supporting leg on the ground slightly away from the bench but at the level of the hip joint.
- Fully extend the arm holding the weight with the palm turned inwards.
- Draw the weight toward the hip joint until the upper arm is parallel with the floor.

Awareness points: Keep the head facing down to maintain neutral cervical spine. Maintain a normal lumbar curve at all times.

Safety point: It is advised to only raise the upper arm until parallel with the floor. If the arm is raised any further than this, then it is the trapezius muscle that is responsible. The latissimus muscle is a much stronger muscle than the trapezius, therefore, if a considerable weight is being used, this could compromise the trapezius leading to strain injury.

Alternatives: Lat Pull Down, Seated Row.

Fig. 15.3 (a) and (b): Single Arm Row

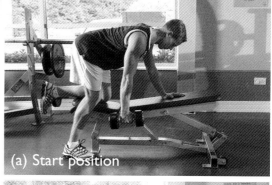

(a) Start position

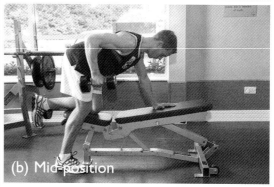

(b) Mid-position

Shoulder Press

Major muscles used: Deltoids (anterior and posterior)

Synergist muscles used: Tricep

Main movement: Abduction of the shoulder/extension of the elbow

- Stand with feet shoulder width apart and the spine in neutral position. Ensure upper arms are slightly below parallel position, with hands directly above the elbow joint.
- The palms should be facing forwards and in line with the front of the face.
- Raise the weights in an arcing motion keeping them in line with the front of the face until the arms are fully extended.

Awareness points: Both hands should remain within peripheral vision at all times. Maintain a normal lumbar curve at all times.

Safety points: Keeping the hands in peripheral vision reduces the risk of impingement injury. Also, if the upper arms are quite far below parallel at the start position, then injury could occur to the supraspinatus muscle as this would be responsible for initiating the movement.

Alternatives: Machine Shoulder Press, Lateral Raise, Upright Row.

Fig. 15.4 **(a) and (b): Shoulder Press**

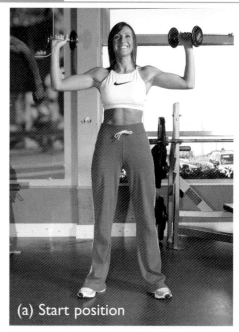

(a) Start position

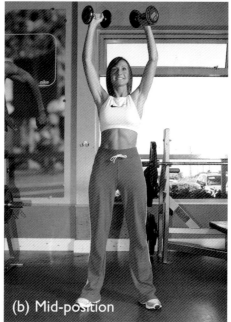

(b) Mid-position

Lateral Raise

Major muscles used: Deltoids (anterior and posterior)

Synergist muscles used: Trapezius (upper fibres during shoulder elevation)

Main movement: Abduction of the shoulder

- Stand with feet shoulder width apart and the spine in neutral position. Hang the arms by the sides with a slight bend at the elbow joint so that the weight is slightly forward of the hip joint, palms facing inwards.
- Raise the weights in an abduction motion keeping them in line and slightly forward of the hip joint until the arms are parallel to the floor.

Awareness points: Both hands should remain within peripheral vision at all times. Maintain a normal lumbar curve at all times. Stop when the upper arms are parallel to the floor.

Safety point: It is advised to stop the movement when the arms are parallel to the floor in order to reduce the risk of impingement with the humerus and acromion process. Also, when going beyond this point it becomes a trapezius exercise, therefore, it is best to perform a specific trapezius exercise such as a shoulder shrug.

Alternatives: Shoulder Press, Upright Row.

Fig. 15.5 (a) and (b): Lateral Raise

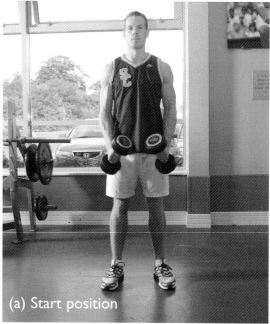

(a) Start position

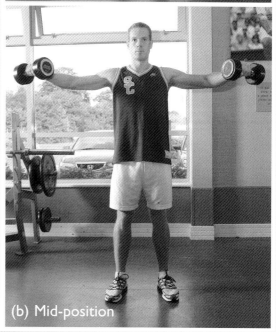

(b) Mid-position

Upright Row

Major muscles used: Deltoids (anterior and posterior)

Synergist muscles used: Trapezius (upper fibres during shoulder elevation), Bicep brachialis

Main movement: Abduction of the shoulder/flexion of the elbow/elevation of the shoulder girdle

- Stand with feet shoulder width apart and the spine in neutral position. Hang the arms to the front of the body with a slight bend at the elbow joint, palms facing inwards.
- Raise the weights in a vertical motion keeping them in front of the body until the upper arms are parallel to the floor.

Awareness points: Maintain a normal lumbar curve at all times. Stop when the upper arms are parallel to the floor.

Safety point: This is similar to the lateral raise in that when the upper arm goes above parallel to the floor it is the trapezius that becomes the prime mover. However, it is often the case that there is an increased risk of injury due to the extreme angle at the wrist.

Alternatives: Lateral Raise, Shoulder Press.

Fig. 15.6 **(a) and (b): Upright Row**

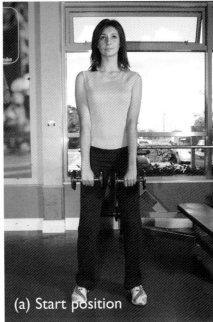

(a) Start position

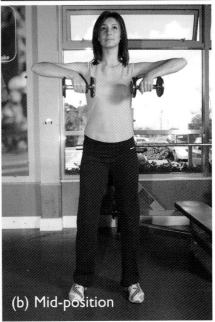

(b) Mid-position

Tricep Extension

Major muscles used: Tricep

Synergist muscles used: Anconeus

Main movement: Extension of the elbow

- Stand with feet shoulder width apart and the spine in neutral position. Extend upper arm directly above the head with a 90 degree bend at the elbow, palm facing inwards.
- Extend the arm so that the hand is directly above the shoulder joint.

Awareness points: Maintain a normal lumbar curve at all times. Make sure that the weight remains to the side of the head at all times.

Safety point: There is always a degree of risk when a weight is above the head, so use caution or choose a safer option such as the kick-back.

Alternatives: Tricep Push, Tricep Kick-back, Narrow-arm Press-up.

Fig. 15.7 **(a) and (b): Tricep Extension**

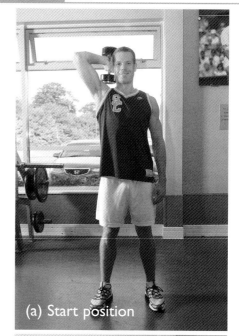

(a) Start position

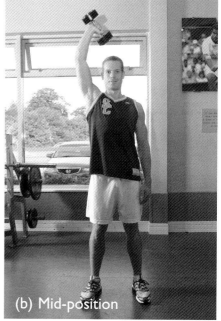

(b) Mid-position

Tricep Kick-Back

Major muscles used: Tricep

Synergist muscles used: Anconeus

Main movement: Extension of the elbow

- Adopt a kneeling position with one leg so that the hip joint of that leg is at approximately 90 degrees and the supporting hand is directly below the shoulder.
- Place the supporting leg on the ground slightly away from the bench but at the level of the hip joint.
- With the palm turned inwards raise the upper arm until it is parallel with the floor and keep a 90-degree angle at the elbow joint.
- Extend the lower arm backwards until it is parallel with the floor.

Awareness points: Keep the head facing down to maintain neutral cervical spine. Maintain a normal lumbar curve at all times. Also, in order to exercise the full range of the tricep, try lowering the upper arm at the end of the movement so that it is below parallel as the tricep crosses the shoulder joint and performs shoulder extension.

Safety points: Try to keep the head facing the floor as there is a tendency to look up and rotate the head to look at the weight which can cause unnecessary pressure on the cervical region.

Alternatives: Tricep Push, Tricep Extension, Narrow-arm Press-up.

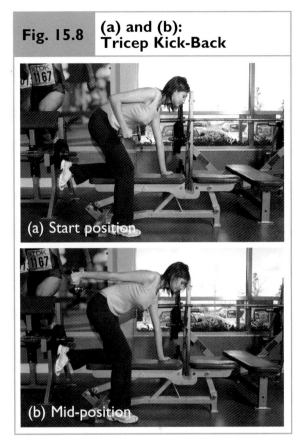

Fig. 15.8 **(a) and (b): Tricep Kick-Back**

(a) Start position

(b) Mid-position

Bicep Curl

Major muscles used: Biceps brachii

Synergist muscles used: Bicep brachialis, brachioradialis

Main movement: Flexion of the elbow

- Stand with feet shoulder width apart and the spine in neutral position. Hang the arms by the sides with palms facing forwards.
- Raise the weights in a line towards the face as if feeding.

Awareness points: Maintain a normal lumbar curve at all times. Make sure that the weights do not strike the face and lower them to full extension of the elbow joint.

Safety point: Avoid any twisting motion at the start of the movement as flexion and rotation often lead to tendon problems such as epicondylitis (golfer's or tennis elbow).

Alternatives: Bicep Curl Machine.

Fig. 15.9 **(a) and (b): Bicep Curl**

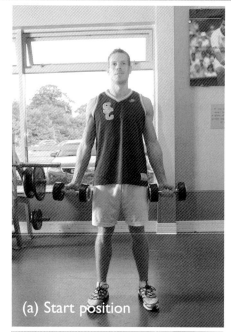

(a) Start position

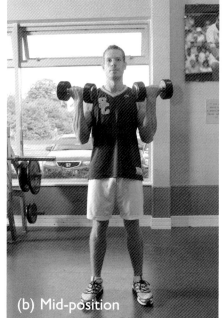

(b) Mid-position

Squat

Major muscles used: Quadriceps (vastus lateralis, vastus medialis, vastus intermedius, rectus femoris), hamstrings (bicep femoris, semitendonosus, semimembranosus), gluteus maximus, erector spinae

Synergist muscles used: Some of the muscles above work as synergists depending on the angle of the torso

Main movement: Extension of the spine, hip, knee and ankle

- Stand with feet shoulder width apart and the spine in neutral position. Hang the arms by the sides with palms facing inwards.
- Bend the hip joint and knee joint as in a sitting motion until the individual is at their full range.

Awareness points: Maintain a normal lumbar curve at all times. The head should drop and raise in a vertical line so that the body does not tilt forward.

Safety point: Always encourage individuals to squat through their full range as limiting the range of motion can lead to weakness (and lack of flexibility) at certain points in the range of the movement.

Alternatives: Squat Machine

Fig. 15.10 (a) and (b): Squat

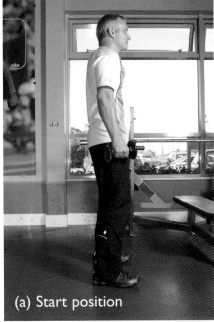

(a) Start position

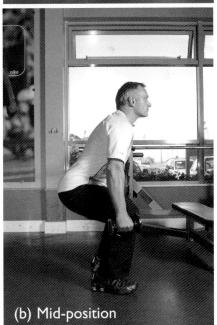

(b) Mid-position

Chest Press

Major muscles used: Pectoralis major

Synergist muscles used: Anterior deltoid, tricep, serratus anterior

Main movement: Horizontal adduction of the shoulder/elbow extension

- Make sure the feet are placed firmly on the ground and that the seat is at the height where the arms are parallel to the floor.
- The upper arms should be in line with the body.
- Fully extend the arms, keeping the wrists firm.

Awareness points: Maintain a normal lumbar curve at all times. Do not allow the hands to go out of peripheral vision at any time.

Safety points: Most machines allow a starting point where the upper arms are further back than the line of the body. This can place too much strain on the anterior deltoid (as in the free-weight version). Set the machine so that the shoulder joint feels as though it is not on stretch.

Alternatives: Free-weight Chest Press, Chest Flye, Pec Dec, Press-ups.

Fig. 15.11 **(a) and (b): Chest Press**

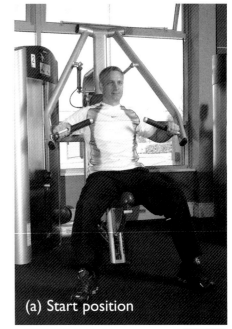

(a) Start position

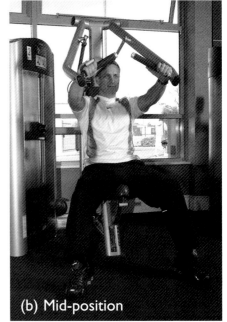

(b) Mid-position

Pec Dec

Major muscles used: Pectoralis major

Synergist muscles used: Anterior deltoid, serratus anterior

Main movement: Horizontal adduction of the shoulder

- Make sure the feet are placed firmly on the ground and that the seat is at the height where the upper arms are parallel to the floor.
- The arms should be in line with the body.
- Bring the arms together under control.

Awareness points: Maintain a normal lumbar curve at all times. Do not allow the hands to go out of peripheral vision at any time.

Safety point: Most pec decs are set up so that the upper arm is laterally rotated in order to place the hands on the pads. This has the effect of wrapping the pectoral tendon over the humerus. In order to avoid this, try doing the exercise with straight arms so that the hands are not on the pads. This will put the pectoral tendon in the right place.

Alternatives: Chest Press, Chest Flye, Press-ups.

Fig. 15.12 **(a) and (b): Pec Dec**

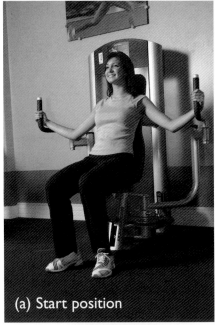

(a) Start position

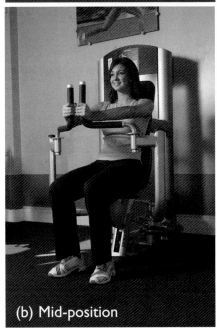

(b) Mid-position

Shoulder Press

Major muscles used: Deltoids (anterior and posterior)

Synergist muscles used: Tricep

Main movement: Adduction of the shoulder/extension of the elbow

- Make sure feet are firmly on the ground and the spine is in neutral position. Adjust the seat height until the upper arms are slightly below parallel position.
- Raise the arms until they are fully extended.

Awareness points: Both hands should remain within peripheral vision at all times. Maintain a normal lumbar curve at all times.

Safety points: Keeping the hands in peripheral vision reduces the risk of impingement injury. Also, if the upper arms are quite far below parallel at the start position, then injury could occur to the supraspinatus muscle as this would be responsible for initiating the movement.

Alternatives: Free-weight Shoulder Press, Lateral Raise, Upright Row.

Fig. 15.13 (a) and (b): Shoulder Press

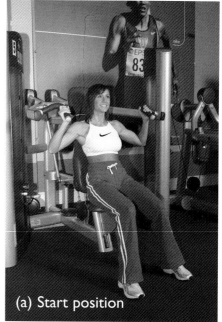

(a) Start position

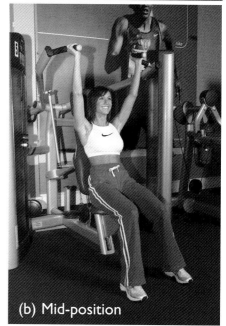

(b) Mid-position

Seated Row

Major muscles used: Latissimus dorsi

Synergist muscles used: Bicep brachialis, posterior deltoid

Main movement: Extension of the shoulder/ flexion of the elbow

- Make sure the feet are firmly on the floor and the spine is in a neutral position.
- The chest support should be adjusted so that the hands can take a firm grip of the handles with the chest on the support.
- Adjust the seat height so that the arms are roughly parallel to the floor.
- Draw the weight toward the body until the upper arm is parallel with the plane of the body.

Awareness points: Keep the head facing forward to maintain neutral cervical spine. Maintain a normal lumbar curve at all times. Only draw the upper arms back to the plane of the body to avoid undue strain on the trapezius muscle.

Safety point: Limit the movement so that the arms finish parallel to the body. If they pull further back, this will increase the risk of injury to the trapezius as it will be the muscle responsible for this further movement.

Alternatives: Lat Pull-down, Single-arm Row.

Fig. 15.14	(a) and (b): Seated Row

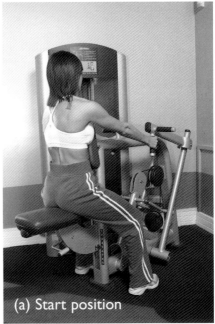

(a) Start position

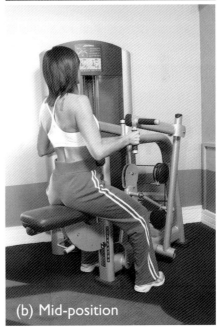

(b) Mid-position

Lat Pull-Down

Major muscles used: Latissimus dorsi

Synergist muscles used: Bicep brachialis, posterior deltoid

Main movement: Adduction of the shoulder/ flexion of the elbow

- Make sure the feet are firmly on the floor and the spine is in a neutral position.
- Adjust the seat height so that the arms are almost at full extension when gripping the handles on the bar.
- Draw the bar vertically down in front of the body until it is roughly in line with the chin level.

Awareness points: Keep the head facing forward to maintain neutral cervical spine. Maintain a normal lumbar curve at all times.

Safety points: Only draw the bar to chin level to avoid undue strain on the rotator cuff muscles as the shoulder would have to internally rotate to go any further. Also, draw the bar to the front of the body to keep the hands in peripheral vision in order to reduce the risk of impingement at the shoulder joints.

Alternatives: Seated Row, Single-arm Row.

Fig. 15.15 **(a) and (b): Lat Pull-Down**

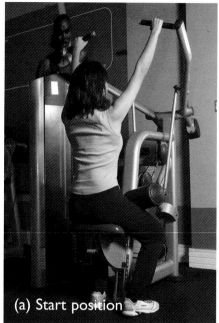

(a) Start position

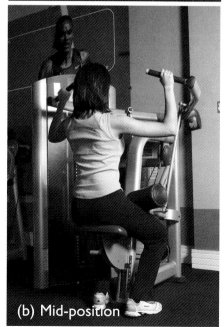

(b) Mid-position

Back Extension

Major muscles used: Most of the erector spinae group of muscles

Synergist muscles used: Multifidus and some of the many individual muscles that make up the erector spinae group

Main movement: Extension of the spine

- Make sure the feet are firmly on the floor or foot plate and the spine is in neutral position.
- Place the pad across the shoulder level with the torso in a flexed position.
- Extend the back to a position where the spine is in neutral.

Awareness points: Keep the head facing forward to maintain neutral cervical spine. Maintain a normal lumbar curve at all times. Avoid going into extension of the spine.

Safety point: The main role of the erector spinae muscle group is to maintain an upright posture whenever we are in a standing position, therefore, limit the extension (but have a full flexion range) to where the body would be in a vertical position rather than a 'lean back' position.

Alternatives: Free-weight Squat, Dorsal Raise.

Fig. 15.16 **(a) and (b): Back Extension**

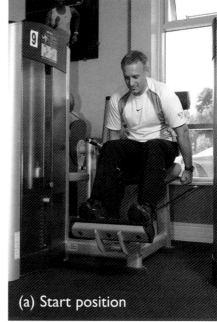

(a) Start position

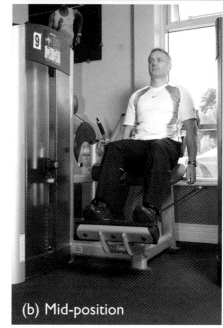

(b) Mid-position

Abdominal Crunch

Major muscles used: Rectus abdominis

Synergist muscles used: Hip flexors (Iliopsoas), external and internal obliques.

Main movement: Flexion of the spine

- Make sure the feet are firmly on the floor or foot plate and the spine is in a neutral position.
- Place the pad across the upper chest.
- Draw the torso towards the knees.

Awareness points: Keep the head facing forward to maintain neutral cervical spine. Maintain a normal lumbar curve at all times.

Safety point: The rectus abdominis is essentially a fast-twitch muscle used for running and jumping, explosive movements, therefore, limit the flexion range or chose an option such as knee lifts.

Alternatives: Knee lifts, Sit-ups, Crunches.

Fig. 15.17 **(a) and (b): Abdominal Crunch**

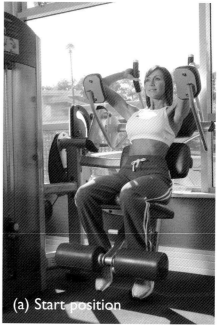

(a) Start position

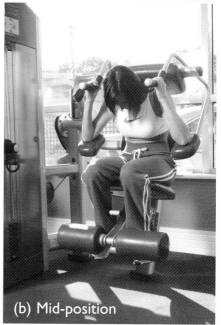

(b) Mid-position

Tricep Push

Major muscles used: Tricep

Synergist muscles used: Anconeus

Main movement: Extension of the elbow

- Make sure the feet are shoulder width apart and the spine is in a neutral position. Grip the bar shoulder width apart so that the upper arms are just forward of the body line, palm facing downwards.
- Extend the upper and lower arm so that the arms are both fully straight.

Awareness points: Maintain a normal lumbar curve at all times.

Safety point: Make sure that there is some shoulder extension in the movement in order to work the full range of the tricep in a functional role.

Alternatives: Tricep Extension, Tricep Kick-back, Narrow-arm Press-up.

Fig. 15.18 | **(a) and (b): Tricep Push**

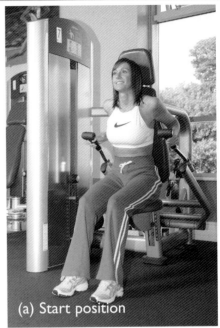

(a) Start position

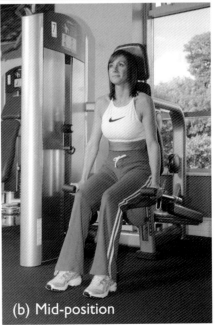

(b) Mid-position

Bicep Curl

Major muscles used: Bicep brachii

Synergist muscles used: Bicep brachialis, brachioradialis

Main movement: Flexion of the elbow

- Make sure the feet are shoulder width apart and the spine is in a neutral position. Grip the handles so that the upper arms are on the pads and the palms face upwards.
- Bring the handles towards the face until the elbow joint is fully flexed.

Awareness points: Maintain a normal lumbar curve at all times. Keep the upper arms on the pad at all times. Fully extend the arms on the downward phase.

Safety point: Try and position the elbow joint directly in line with the pivot of the machine so that the upper arm follows the arc of the machine handles.

Alternatives: Free-weight Bicep Curl.

Fig. 15.19 (a) and (b): Bicep Curl

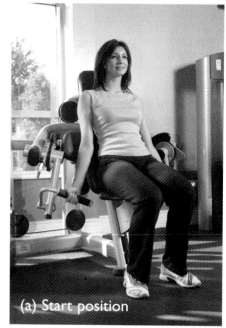

(a) Start position

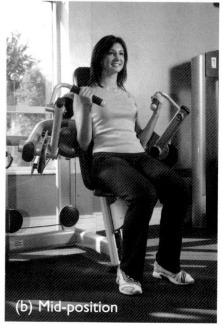

(b) Mid-position

Seated Adductor

Major muscles used: Adductor longus, brevis and magnus, gracilis, pectinius

Main movement: Adduction of the hip

- Ensure the feet are firmly on the foot plates and the pads are on the inside of the knees.
- Use the machine setting to open the legs to a comfortable start position.
- Bring the legs together against the resistance.

Awareness points: Maintain a normal lumbar curve at all times. Keep the knees and the toes pointing directly upwards at all times.

Safety point: The main role of the hip adductors is to stabilise the hip when running and walking, therefore, limit the weight and increase the reps to increase muscular endurance.

Alternatives: Squats, Leg Press, Lunges, Multi-hip Machine.

| Fig. 15.20 | (a) and (b): Seated Adductor |

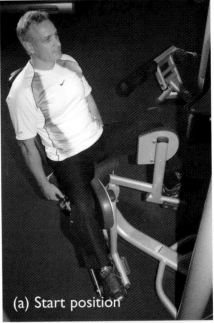

(a) Start position

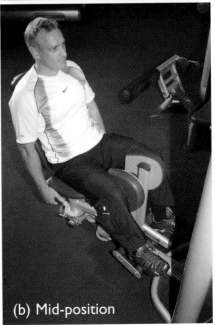

(b) Mid-position

Seated Abductor

Major muscles used: Gluteus minimus and maximus, tensor fascia latae

Synergist muscles used: Sartorius, piriformis

Main movement: Abduction of the hip

- Make sure the feet are firmly on the foot plates and the pads are on the outside of the knees.
- Use the machine setting to start with the legs together.
- Open the legs outwards against the resistance.

Awareness points: Maintain a normal lumbar curve at all times. Open the legs to a full range of motion.

Safety point: The main role of the hip adductors is to stabilise the hip when running and walking, therefore, limit the weight and increase the reps to increase muscular endurance.

Alternatives: Squats, Leg Press, Lunges, Multi-hip Machine.

Fig. 15.21 **(a) and (b): Seated Abductor**

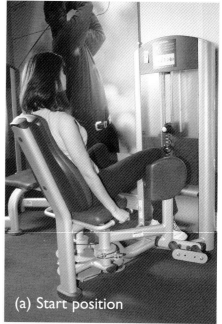

(a) Start position

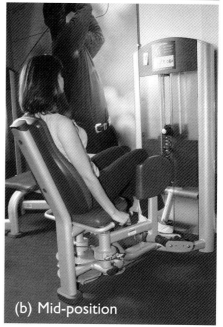

(b) Mid-position

Leg Extension

Major muscles used: Quadriceps (vastus lateralis, vastus medialis, vastus intermedius, rectus femoris)

Main movement: Extension of the knee

- Place the roller pads just above the ankle joint.
- Use the machine seat-setting to move the seat so that the knee joint is just at the edge of the seat.
- Start with the knees flexed as far as comfortably possible.
- Extend the knees to full range of motion.

Awareness points: Maintain a normal lumbar curve at all times. Keep the knees and the toes pointing directly upwards at all times. Ensure that full extension is achieved.

Safety point: Not going to full extension can result in weakness of the vastus medialis muscle (one of the quads), which only fully contracts in the last few degrees of the movement. If this weakens, it could result in patella mall tracking (where the patella does not run in the groove at the end of the femur) and erosion of the articular cartilage on the underside of the patella.

Alternatives: Squats, Leg Press, Lunges.

Fig. 15.22	(a) and (b): Leg Extension

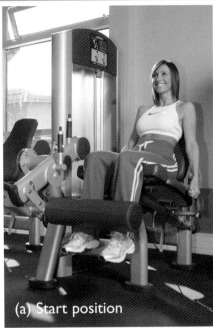

(a) Start position

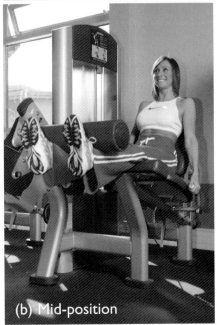

(b) Mid-position

Leg Curl

Major muscles used: Hamstrings (bicep femoris, semitendonosus, semimembranosus)

Synergist muscles used: Calf (gastrocnemius and soleus)

Main movement: Flexion of the knee

- Place the roller pads just above the calcaneus or heel bone.
- Use the machine seat-setting to move the seat so that the knee joint is just at the edge of the seat.
- Start with the knees extended as far as comfortably possible.
- Flex the knees to full range of motion.

Awareness points: Maintain a normal lumbar curve at all times. Keep the knees and the toes pointing directly upwards at all times.

Safety points: The main function of the hamstrings is during walking and running when the thigh comes forward (hip flexion) at the same time as the hamstrings contract during knee flexion. If the machine has a pad that comes down on the thighs, try not to use it if possible as this would restrict movement of the thigh, which is what the body is normally used to.

Alternatives: Squats, Leg Press, Lunges.

Fig. 15.23 (a) and (b): Leg Curl

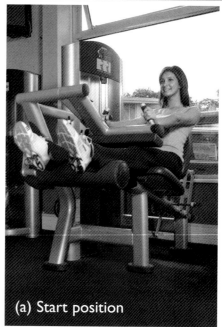

(a) Start position

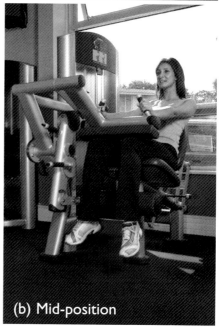

(b) Mid-position

Leg Press

Major muscles used: Quadriceps (vastus lateralis, vastus medialis, vastus intermedius, rectus femoris), hamstrings (bicep femoris, semitendonosus, semimembranosus), gluteus maximus

Synergist muscles used: Some of the muscles above work as synergists depending on the foot placement

Main movement: Extension of the hip, knee and ankle

- Place the feet about hip-width apart on the foot plate.
- Use the machine seat-setting to move the seat so that the knee joint is flexed to the maximum comfortable position.
- Extend the knees to full range of motion.

Awareness points: Maintain a normal lumbar curve at all times. Keep the knees and the toes in line at all times. Ensure that full extension at the knee joint is achieved.

Safety point: Do not limit the movement to approximately 90 degrees. All individuals should be encouraged to have a full range of movement in order to strengthen at the outer range and help flexibility which is often lacking.

Alternatives: Squats, Lunges

Fig. 15.24 **(a) and (b): Leg Press**

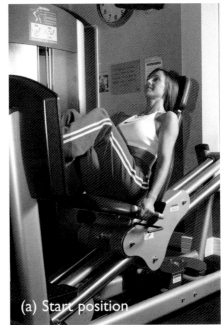

(a) Start position

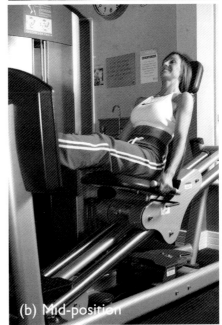

(b) Mid-position

Internal Rotation

Major muscles used: Teres major, subscapularis.

Synergist muscles used: Latissimus dorsi, pectoralis major, anterior deltoid.

Main movement: Internal rotation of the shoulder

- Stand with feet shoulder width apart and the spine in neutral position. Hold the cable so that the forearm is parallel to the ground and fully externally rotated.
- Bring the forearm across the body.

Awareness points: Maintain a normal lumbar curve at all times. The forearm should remain parallel to the floor throughout the movement. Adjust the tension on the band to suit if not using a cable.

Safety point: Shoulder stabilisers tend to be weak so encourage lighter weights.

Alternatives: Use a flexi-tube or resistance band anchored to a suitable machine at elbow height.

Fig. 15.25 **(a) and (b): Internal Rotation**

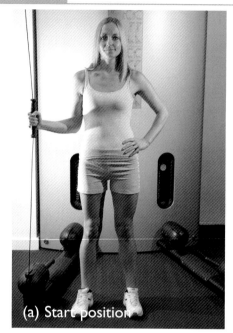

(a) Start position

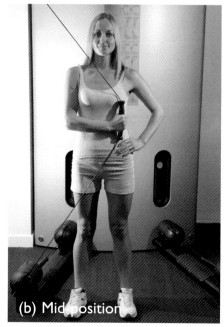

(b) Mid position

External Rotation

Major muscles used: Teres minor, infraspinatus.

Synergist muscles used: Posterior deltoid.

Main movement: External rotation of the shoulder

- Stand with feet shoulder width apart and the spine in neutral position. Hold the cable so that the forearm is parallel to the ground and fully internally rotated.
- Take the forearm across and away from the body.

Awareness points: Maintain a normal lumbar curve at all times. The forearm should remain parallel to the floor throughout the movement. Adjust the tension on the band to suit if not using a cable.

Safety point: Shoulder stabilisers tend to be weak so encourage lighter weights.

Alternatives: Use a flexi-tube or resistance band anchored to a suitable machine at elbow height.

Fig. 15.26 | **(a) and (b): External Rotation**

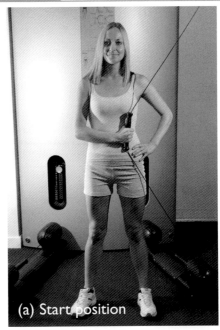

(a) Start position

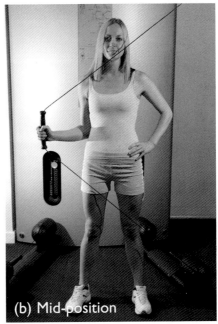

(b) Mid-position

EXAMPLE QUESTIONS: ANSWERS FOR REVISION

I THE SKELETAL SYSTEM

1.1 The radius bone is an example of which type of bone?
  a) long bone

1.2 The patella is an example of which type of bone?
  d) sesamoid bone

1.3 The scapula is an example of which type of bone?
  c) flat bone

1.4 What is the name for the area near the end of a long bone where growth occurs?
  b) epiphysis

1.5 Which two regions of the spine are secondary curves?
  c) lumbar and cervical

1.6 In which region of the spine are the bones fused?
  d) sacrum

1.7 Tendons attach to a layer of tissue covering a bone. What is this covering called?
  d) periostium

1.8 Cells in the bone that are responsible for bone-building are called what?
  b) osteoblast cells

1.9 Cells in the bone that are responsible for breaking down bone are called what?
  c) osteoclast cells

1.10 In terms of postural deviation, an excessive primary curve of the thoracic region of the spine is usually referred to by what name?
  d) kyphosis

EXAMPLE QUESTIONS: ANSWERS FOR REVISION cont.

1.11 In terms of postural deviation, an excessive secondary curve of the lumbar region of the spine is usually referred to by what name?

a) lordosis

1.12 In terms of postural deviation, twisting of the spine is usually referred to by what name?

b) scoliosis

2 JOINTS

2.1 The tibia and the fibula make what type of joint?

a) fixed

2.2 The facet joints of the transverse processes of the spine make what type of joint?

a) cartilaginous

2.3 The tibia and the femur make what type of joint?

c) synovial

2.4 The pubis symphysis is what type of joint?

b) cartilaginous

2.5 Which of the following is classed as a hinge joint?

c) elbow

2.6 Which two movements are available at a saddle joint?

b) flexion, extension, adduction and abduction

2.7 Which of the following make a joint?

c) femur and pelvis

EXAMPLE QUESTIONS: ANSWERS FOR REVISION cont.

2.8 Which of the following make a joint?
b) humerus and scapula

2.9 Which of the following make a joint?
a) metacarpals and phalanges

2.10 Which of the following make a joint?
a) tarsals and tibia

2.11 Which of the following make a gliding joint?
c) bones of the carpals

2.12 Which of the following make a pivot joint?
b) atlas and axis

3 THE MUSCULAR SYSTEM

3.1 What is the main fuel of type I fibres?
a) fat and oxygen

3.2 What is the main fuel of type IIb fibres?
c) glucose

3.3 Which type of muscle can be found in the digestive system?
d) smooth

3.4 Which type of muscle can be found in the heart?
b) cardiac

3.5 In muscle contraction, which hormone is released from the end motor plate and crosses the synaptic gap?
b) acetyl choline

EXAMPLE QUESTIONS: ANSWERS FOR REVISION cont.

3.6 Which term is used to describe a muscle under tension where the origin and insertion move away from each other?

   c) eccentric

3.7 Which term is used to describe a muscle under tension where the origin and insertion move closer together?

   b) concentric

3.8 What is the name given to a muscle when performing the role of stabilising a joint?

   d) fixator

3.9 What is the name given to a muscle when performing the role of assisting the agonist muscle?

   c) synergist

3.10 What is the name given to a muscle when performing the main action?

   a) agonist

3.11 Which exercise is associated with the sagittal plane?

   d) leg extension

3.12 Which exercise is associated with the frontal or coronal plane?

   c) pull down

4 CARTILAGE, LIGAMENT AND TENDON

4.1 What type of cartilage can be described as a thin, tough, shiny, bluey-white membrane?

   c) articular

EXAMPLE QUESTIONS: ANSWERS FOR REVISION cont.

4.2 What type of cartilage can be described as bundles of fibres that provide flexible support?

b) elastic

4.3 What type of cartilage can be described as a thick, strong and spongy shock-absorber?

a) fibro

4.4 What is fibro cartilage mainly made up of?

b) collagen

4.5 Which is a ligament of the knee?

c) lateral collateral

4.6 Which is a ligament of the shoulder?

c) coracohumeral

4.7 Which is a ligament of the hip?

a) ischiofemoral

4.8 Which is a ligament of the ankle?

b) calcaneotibial

4.9 Which type of tissue connects bone to bone?

c) ligament

4.10 Which type of tissue connects muscle to bone?

b) tendon

4.11 What is the name of the fibro cartilage in the knee joint?

d) meniscus

EXAMPLE QUESTIONS: ANSWERS FOR REVISION cont.

4.12 Which type of tissue does the statement 'allows wanted but prevents unwanted movement' relate to?

c) ligament

5 NERVOUS AND ENDOCRINE SYSTEMS

5.1 Glands are responsible for secreting what into the bloodstream?

c) hormones

5.2 Nerve endings are responsible for secreting what?

a) neurotransmitters

5.3 Nerves that lead away from the central nervous system are known as what?

b) motor or efferent

5.4 Nerves that lead back to the central nervous system are known as what?

a) sensory or afferent

5.5 Which of the following receptors sense position?

a) proprioceptors

5.6 Which of the following receptors sense pain?

c) nociceptors

5.7 Which of the following receptors sense temperature?

d) thermoreceptors

5.8 Which of the following receptors sense chemical composition?

b) chemoreceptors

5.9 Catecholamines and corticosteroids are secreted by which gland?

d) adrenals

EXAMPLE QUESTIONS: ANSWERS FOR REVISION cont.

5.10 Tyrosine based hormones that regulate metabolism are secreted by which gland?
  b) thyroid

5.11 Glucagon is secreted by which gland?
  c) pancreas

5.12 Testosterone and oestrogen are secreted by which gland?
  d) testes and ovaries

6 ENERGY SYSTEMS

6.1 When a phosphate molecule is split from ATP what does it leave?
  d) ADP

6.2 What is the main process that occurs within mitochondria?
  b) production of ATP in the presence of oxygen

6.3 Anaerobic glycolysis is…
  b) breaking down glucose without the presence of oxygen

6.4 Aerobic glycolysis is…
  a) breaking down glucose in the presence of oxygen

6.5 Which of the following is given off as a by-product of aerobic glycolysis?
  d) carbon dioxide and water

6.6 Which of the following is given off as a by-product of anaerobic glycolysis?
  c) lactic acid

6.7 Which of the following is produced as a result of incomplete breakdown of fat due to lack of available carbohydrate?
  c) ketones

EXAMPLE QUESTIONS: ANSWERS FOR REVISION cont.

6.8 Which energy system contributes the most (in percentage terms) at the start of exercise?

c) ATP-PC system

6.9 Which energy system contributes the least (in percentage terms) at the start of exercise?

d) aerobic (fat)

6.10 Which energy system contributes the most (in percentage terms) in short sprint events such as the 100 metres?

c) ATP-PC system

6.11 Which energy system contributes the most (in percentage terms) in events such as the 800 metres?

b) aerobic glycolysis

6.12 Which energy system contributes the most (in percentage terms) in events such as a long distance run?

b) aerobic (fat)

7 THE HEART AND THE CIRCULATORY SYSTEM

7.1 The heart muscle is divided into left and right sides by what?

d) septum

7.2 The heart muscle is entirely covered by a layer of fibrous tissue known as what?

a) pericardium

7.3 The term 'entry hall' relates to which structure in the heart?

c) atrium

EXAMPLE QUESTIONS: ANSWERS FOR REVISION cont.

7.4 The mitral valve is otherwise known as the what?
c) bi-cuspid

7.5 The sino-atrial node can be found in which chamber of the heart?
a) right atrium

7.6 The aortic valve can be found leading from which chamber of the heart?
d) left ventricle

7.7 The amount of blood pumped out of the ventricles each beat is known as what?
c) stroke volume

7.8 The amount of blood pumped out of the ventricles each beat, multiplied by the heart rate in beats per minute is known as what?
b) cardiac output

7.9 The amount of blood left in the ventricles after each beat is known as what?
a) end diastolic volume

7.10 Which of the following protect the body against foreign bodies?
a) white blood cells

7.11 Which of the following help in blood clotting?
b) platelets

7.12 Blood pressure is greatest in which vessel?
c) aorta

8 THE RESPIRATORY SYSTEM

8.1 What structures lead directly into the alveoli?
a) bronchioles

EXAMPLE QUESTIONS: ANSWERS FOR REVISION cont.

8.2 The double membrane surrounding the lungs is known as what?

b) pleura

8.6 The passage of oxygen and carbon dioxide in and out of the alveoli is known as what?

a) gaseous exchange

8.4 What is the percentage of oxygen in the air that is inspired?

c) 21

8.5 The amount of air left in the lungs after a breath out is known as what?

c) residual volume

8.6 The maximum amount of air breathed out of the lungs after a maximum breath in is known as what?

d) vital capacity

8.7 Which of the following gases stimulates breathing when blood levels reach a certain point?

b) carbon dioxide

8.8 The amount of air taken into the lungs during a normal breath is called what?

b) tidal volume

8.9 Smoking is thought to be one of the main causes of what?

a) chronic bronchitis

8.10 Inflammation of the alveoli is otherwise known as what?

c) pneumonia

8.11 Normal expiration is brought about as a result of what effect?

d) elastic recoil

EXAMPLE QUESTIONS: ANSWERS FOR REVISION cont.

8.12 Which is the main muscle involved in forced expiration?

d) transversus abdominis

9 CORE STABILITY

9.1 Which of the following properties relates to stabilising muscles?

d) postural, endurance, tonic, slow twitch

9.2 Which of the following properties relates to mobilising muscles?

c) short-term, explosive, phasic, fast twitch

9.3 Which of the following can be considered to be predominantly stabilising muscles for the core?

b) multifidus, transversus abdominis, pelvic floor

9.4 Which of the following can be considered to be predominantly mobilising muscles for the core?

c) erector spinae, external oblique, rectus abdominus

9.5 Which of the following can be considered to be a predominantly stabilising muscle for the hip joint?

d) gluteus medius

9.6 Which of the following can be considered to be predominantly a mobilising muscle for the hip joint?

b) gluteus maximus

9.7 When local muscles contract to compress the 'fluid ball' in the abdomen it is known as what?

b) intra-abdominal pressure

EXAMPLE QUESTIONS: ANSWERS FOR REVISION cont.

9.8 An increase in the tension of the connective tissues in the spinal region is known as what?

d) thoraco-lumbar fascia gain

9.9 Research has suggested that what percentage of maximum contraction is sufficient to create sufficient intra-abdominal pressure to stabilise the spine?

d) 30

9.10 What best relates to the statement *'when there is minimal force placed on the spine and the structures that surround it such as tendons, cartilage and ligaments'*?

b) neutral zone

9.11 True or false? Normal screening procedures should be carried out prior to prescribing core stabilisation exercises but those with back problems should be excluded.

True

9.12 The length of time, number of repetitions and frequency of practice of conscious contraction required to develop sub-conscious contraction control of the transversus abdominis can take up to how long?

d) a few months

10 COMPONENTS AND PRINCIPLES OF FITNESS

10.1 The ACSM define what as *'an ability to perform daily activities with vigour and the demonstration of traits and capacities that are associated with a low risk of premature development of hypokinetic diseases'*?

c) health related physical fitness

10.2 The World Health Organisation defines what as *'a state of complete physical, mental and social well-being and not merely the absence of disease or infirmity'*?

a) wellness

EXAMPLE QUESTIONS: ANSWERS FOR REVISION cont.

10.3 Cardiovascular endurance is also known as what?
b) aerobic capacity

10.4 $mlO_2.kg^{-1}min^{-1}$ is a measurement of what?
c) VO_2max

10.5 What are the benefits of regular cardiovascular training?
a) increased HDL, increased exercise threshold, decreased heart rate for given intensity

10.6 What is the term used to define an increase in muscle cross-section?
c) hypertrophy

10.7 What is the term used to define a decrease in muscle cross-section?
b) atrophy

10.8 What are the benefits of regular resistance training?
a) increased glucose tolerance, increased bone mass, increased resting metabolic rate

10.9 Strength gains in the first few weeks of a resistance training programme are usually due to what?
d) neural changes

10.10 What type of stretching involves the contraction of the agonist to elicit a stretch in the antagonist?
b) dynamic

10.11 Which of the following formulae can be used to calculate BMI?
b) weight/height^2

10.12 In relation to BMI, what figure is classed as obese?
b) over 30

EXAMPLE QUESTIONS: ANSWERS FOR REVISION cont.

11 SCREENING FOR EXERCISE AND SAFETY ISSUES

11.1 The PAR-Q is a screening questionnaire used to identify conditions prior to encouraging exercise at...
   c) a light to moderate intensity

11.2 The PAR-Q is a screening questionnaire which is valid for what period of time?
   d) 12 months

11.3 True or false? The PAR-Q is a confidential document.
   True

11.4 Which of the following is classed as a risk factor in relation to 'family history'?
   b) Myocardial Infarction (MI) or sudden death before age 55 in father, brother or son. Before age 65 in mother, sister or daughter.

11.5 Which of the following is classed as a risk factor in relation to 'hypertension'?
   d) Systolic pressure of 140mmhg or above, or diastolic of 90mmhg or above.

11.6 Which of the following is classed as a risk factor in relation to 'obesity'?
   d) Body Mass Index of 30kg/m^2 or above.

11.7 Which of the following is classed as a risk factor in relation to 'dyslipidemia'?
   c) Total serum cholesterol of more than 5.2mmol/L

11.8 Which of the following is classed as a risk factor in relation to 'dyslipidemia'?
   a) LDL more than 3.4mmol/L, or HDL less than 1.03mmol/L

11.9 With regards to risk stratification, the ACSM state that people who are at moderate risk are...
   c) Men 45 years or older and women 55 years or older or those with two or more risk factors.

EXAMPLE QUESTIONS: ANSWERS FOR REVISION cont.

11.10 Which of the following is classed as a risk factor in relation to 'impaired fasting glucose'?
c) 100mg/dL or more.

11.11 The Health and Safety at Work Act (HSWA) 1974 outlines which of the following as roles of the instructor?
c) both A and B

11.12 True or false? The Health and Safety (First Aid) Regulations 1981 states that employers provide adequate equipment and facilities to enable first aid to be carried out on employees but not necessarily customers using the facility.
True

12 BEHAVIOURAL CHANGE AND GOAL SETTING

12.1 The 'stages of change' model follows what type of pattern?
b) cyclical

12.2 Approximately what percentage of all individuals will experience relapse back to the contemplation or pre-contemplation stage?
c) 15%

12.3 True or false? Cognitive processes are usually adopted by individuals in the early stages of the 'stages of change model' from not thinking about exercise to the action of taking up exercise.
True

12.4 True or false? Behavioural processes are usually adopted by individuals in the later stages of the 'stages of change model'.
True

EXAMPLE QUESTIONS: ANSWERS FOR REVISION cont.

12.5 What is the following a definition of? *'The internal mechanisms and external stimuli which arouse and direct our behaviour'.*
d) motivation

12.6 Which term is used to describe when an individual is motivated to exercise by factors such as enjoyment, fun or self-satisfaction?
a) intrinsic motivation

12.7 When a skill is broken down into manageable units that the subject can focus on, it is otherwise known as what type of goal?
c) process

12.8 The World Health Organization suggests an average daily intake of carbohydrate, fat and protein for the general population should be made up of which of the following?
b) 30% fat, 10–15% protein, 55–60% carbohydrates

12.9 Which of the following vitamins is considered to be important for promoting calcium absorption from food?
c) D

12.10 Which of the following vitamins is considered to be important for producing blood clotting proteins?
b) K

12.11 Which of the following minerals is considered to be important for brain and nerve function?
b) potassium

12.12 Which of the following minerals is considered to be important for the regulation of body water content and nerve function?
a) sodium

EXAMPLE QUESTIONS: ANSWERS FOR REVISION cont.

13 COMPONENTS AND INDUCTION OF AN EXERCISE SESSION

13.1 According to research what is considered to be the main factor in muscular injury prevention?

b) muscle temperature

13.2 In terms of cardiovascular training at the end of the warm-up the heart rate should be at what level?

c) that required for the cardiovascular session to follow

13.3 In relation to cardio training zones, what range of heart range maximum is the 'weight management zone'?

b) 60–70%

13.4 In relation to cardio training zones, what range of heart range maximum is the 'aerobic zone'?

c) 70–80%

13.5 Which of the following are considered to be the main benefits of cardiovascular training?

d) increased fat metabolism, increased glycogen stores, increased aerobic and anaerobic enzymes, increased number and size of mitochondria

13.6 What type of training is otherwise known as 'speed play'?

d) Fartlek

13.7 Which cycle of periodisation is usually associated with a 7-day period?

b) microcycle

13.8 Which cycle of periodisation is usually associated with a period of a few weeks?

c) mesocycle

EXAMPLE QUESTIONS: ANSWERS FOR REVISION cont.

13.9 Which cycle of periodisation is usually associated with a 12-month period?
d) macrocycle

13.10 The ACSM guidelines for stretching suggest holding the stretch for what period of time?
b) 15–30 seconds

13.11 The acronym IDEA refers to what?
a) induction for cardiovascular machines

13.12 Which of the following cardiovascular machines is normally associated with higher impact?
c) treadmill

14 MONITORING EXERCISE INTENSITY

14.1 What is the formula for predicted maximum heart rate?
c) 220 - age

14.2 True or false? Predicted maximum heart rate can have an error of up to plus or minus 12 beats per minute.
True

14.3 True or false? A graded maximum heart rate test should be used on all individuals to find their maximum heart rate.
False

14.4 What is the predicted maximum heart rate for a 29 year old person?
b) 191 bpm

14.5 What is 70% of predicted maximum heart rate for a 40-year-old person?
c) 126 bpm

EXAMPLE QUESTIONS: ANSWERS FOR REVISION cont.

14.6 What is 80% of predicted maximum heart rate for a 20-year-old person?

a) 160 bpm

14.7 What is 55% of predicted maximum heart rate for a 31-year-old person (round up)?

d) 104 bpm

14.8 What is the equivalent value of 2 MET?

c) $7 \text{ mlO}_2.\text{kg}^{-1}\text{min}^{-1}$

14.9 What is the equivalent value of 1 MET?

a) $1.0 \text{ kcal.kg}^{-1}\text{hr}^{-1}$

14.10 How many kilocalories would an 80kg person expend in 30 minutes doing an exercise valued at 5 METs?

d) 400

14.11 How many kilocalories would an 60kg person expend in 2 hours and 30 minutes doing an exercise valued at 4 METs?

c) 600

14.12 Which of the following statements is most accurate in regards to the definition of 12RM?

d) A weight that can be lifted 12 times and not 13 times.

NOTES

NOTES

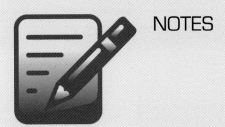

NOTES

APPENDIX: PHYSICAL ACTIVITY GUIDELINES AND CONTRAINDICATIONS FOR ANTENATAL WOMEN

The RCOG and ACOG recommend the following guidelines;

RCOG/ACOG guidelines		
	Aerobic Training	Strength Training
MODE	• Walking, cycling and water based activities are good for this condition.	• Continue as normal if already active. If not, slow progression from body weight to machines / free-weights.
INTENSITY	• RPE level 10-14. • 60-80% HRmax.	• Avoid heavy loads. • Overload by increasing repetitions.
DURATION	• 5-45 minutes per session. • Increase by 2 mins per week but only between the 13th and 28th weeks.	• Perform 1 to 3 sets of 15-20RM. • 1-2 minutes rest between exercises.
FREQUENCY	Active person: • 3-4 per week up to 14th week. • 3-5 per week up to 28th week. • 3 per week after 28th week. Non-active person: • None before 13th week. • 3 per week 13th-36th weeks. • 1-2 per week after 36th week.	• 2-3 sessions per week. • Encourage other forms of exercise. • Decrease weight and sets and increase recovery time as pregnancy progresses.
PRECAUTIONS	• Avoid high impact activities and excessive repetition. • Watch for signs of overheating.	• If no experience prior to pregnancy, do not start. • Avoid overstretching and overhead lifts.

GENERAL PRECAUTIONS:
• Non-active women are advised to seek medical approval BEFORE beginning a programme of activity.
• If any activity causes pain or discomfort, it should be stopped immediately.
• Do rectus abdominis check 6-12 weeks after delivery before doing certain abdominal exercises.
• Be aware of episiotomy and take appropriate steps.
• Avoid motionless standing.
• Avoid supine exercises (lying on the back) after 16 weeks.

Adapted from RCOG guidelines (www.rcog.org.uk/womens-health/clinical-guidance/exercise-pregnancy) and ACOG guidelines (www.acog.org/Search?Keyword=exercise+guidelines).

Contra-indications and reasons to stop activity for pregnant women (RCOG)

Absolute contra-indications to activity

- Haemodynamically significant heart disease
- Restrictive lung disease
- Incompetent cervix/cerclage
- Multiple gestation at risk of preterm labour
- Persistent bleeding in the second and third trimesters
- Placenta praevia after 26 weeks
- Pre-eclampsia or pregnancy-induced hypertension
- Preterm labour (previous/present)
- Preterm rupture of membranes

Relative contraindications to activity

- Severe anaemia (haemoglobin less than 100 g/l).
- Unevaluated maternal cardiac arrhythmia
- Chronic bronchitis
- Poorly controlled type 1 diabetes
- Extreme morbid obesity (BMI > 40)
- Extreme underweight (BMI < 12)
- Extremely sedentary lifestyle
- Intrauterine growth restriction in current pregnancy
- Poorly controlled hypertension/pre-eclampsia
- Orthopaedic limitations
- Poorly controlled thyroid disease
- Poorly controlled seizure disorder
- Heavy smoker (more than 20 cigarettes/day)

Reasons to stop activity

- Excessive shortness of breath
- Chest pain or palpitations
- Presyncope or dizziness
- Painful uterine contractions or preterm labour
- Calf pain or swelling
- Leakage of amniotic fluid
- Vaginal bleeding
- Excessive fatigue
- Abdominal pain, particularly in back or pubic area

- Pelvic girdle pain
- Reduced foetal movement
- Dyspnoea before exertion
- Headache or visual disturbance
- Muscle weakness
- Sudden calf pain or swelling in the ankles, hands or face
- Insufficient weight gain (less than 1 kg per month) - during last two trimesters

Adapted from RCOG guidelines (www.rcog.org.uk/womens-health/clinical-guidance/exercise-pregnancy) and ACOG guidelines (www.acog.org/Search?Keyword=exercise+guidelines).

Even though some of these terms may be unfamiliar, if the intention is to supervise a physical activity programme for someone who is pregnant, these questions should be asked before any activity is undertaken, particularly if they have any of the contra-indications. This shouldn't be a problem as someone who is pregnant should have a good understanding of the terms and be used to answering questions.

APPENDIX: PHYSICAL ACTIVITY GUIDELINES AND CONTRAINDICATIONS FOR OLDER ADULTS

The Department of Health recommends the following exercise guidelines.

DoH guidelines table
1. Older adults who participate in any amount of physical activity gain some health benefits, including maintenance of good physical and cognitive function. Some physical activity is better than none, and more physical activity provides greater health benefits.
2. Older adults should aim to be active daily. Over a week, activity should add up to at least 150 minutes (2½ hours) of moderate intensity activity in bouts of 10 minutes or more – one way to approach this is to do 30 minutes on at least 5 days a week.
3. For those who are already regularly active at moderate intensity, comparable benefits can be achieved through 75 minutes of vigorous intensity activity spread across the week or a combination of moderate and vigorous activity.
4. Older adults should also undertake physical activity to improve muscle strength on at least two days a week.
5. Older adults at risk of falls should incorporate physical activity to improve balance and co-ordination on at least two days a week.
6. All older adults should minimise the amount of time spent being sedentary (sitting) for extended periods

Department of Health, 'Start Active, Stay Active: A report on physical activity for health from the four home counties' chief medical officers', 2011.

There are few absolute contraindications for exercise by older adults, however, there are some that have been suggested such as unstable coronary artery disease or recent myocardial infarction, congestive heart failure that has progressed to dyspnea at rest, tachyarrhythmias induced by activity, and critical aortic stenosis. Non-cardiac contraindications usually include the immediate hypoxic period after a pulmonary emboli, retinal detachment, and unstable cervical spinal conditions. It should be noted however that according to the American College of Sports Medicine, all older adults for whom moderate to vigorous exercise is considered require a screening exercise tolerance test but there are contraindications to testing as shown below.

Absolute and Relative Contraindications to Exercise Testing

Absolute Contraindications	Relative Contraindications
Acute myocardial infarction (within 2 days)	Left main coronary stenosis
Unstable angina	Moderate stenotic valvular heart disease
Uncontrolled cardiac arrhythmias causing symptoms of hemodynamic compromise	Known electrolyte abnormalities (hypokalemia, hypomagnesemia)
Uncontrolled symptomatic heart failure	Mental or physical impairment leading to inability to exercise adequately
Acute aortic dissection	Severe arterial hypertension; resting diastolic BP>110mmHg and/or resting systolic BP > 200 mmHg
Suspected or known dissecting aneurysm	Tachyarrhythmias or bradyarrhythmias
Acute myocarditis or pericarditis	Hypertrophic cardiomyopathy and other forms of outflow tract obstruction
Acute pulmonary embolus or pulmonary infarction	High-degree atrioventricular block

Adapted from the American College of Cardiology and American Heart Association exercise testing guidelines

INDEX

ALSO AVAILABLE IN THE FITNESS PROFESSIONALS SERIES

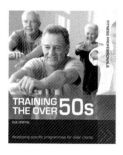

Training the Over 50s

The 50-plus age range has one of the fastest growing groups of regular gym-goers, who are increasingly turning to fitness instructors for guidance. Sue Griffin – a health promotions consultant who specialises in writing education programmes for adults and specialist populations – explains the relationship between fitness and ageing, and gives advice on training adults with chronic conditions and designing individual programmes. Packed with photographs and illustrations, this is the definitive handbook for any fitness professional working with older adults.

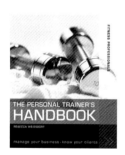

The Personal Trainer's Handbook

Whether you are newly qualified and looking for guidance on setting up your business or an established trainer looking for ideas to develop your company, this book will provide you with all the information you need. Rebecca Weissbort – a practising fitness trainer who has been involved in developing national standards for the fitness industry's governing body – gives invaluable advice on essential business skills, meeting clients' specific needs, and many other aspects of the personal training industry.

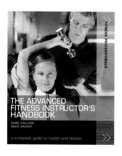

The Advanced Fitness Instructor's Handbook

This is the first book written for the specific needs of fitness professionals studying towards teaching or coaching in one-on-one, group or team situations. Developing key concepts covered in *The Fitness Instructor's Handbook*, this book covers many components of the fitness industry standards for both Level 2 and 3 knowledge requirements. Packed with photos, illustrations and case studies, it offers the perfect blend of theory and practice.

Available from all good bookshops or online. For more details on these and other Bloomsbury sport and fitness titles, please go to www.bloomsbury.com.